Dear Grace,

A Romance of History

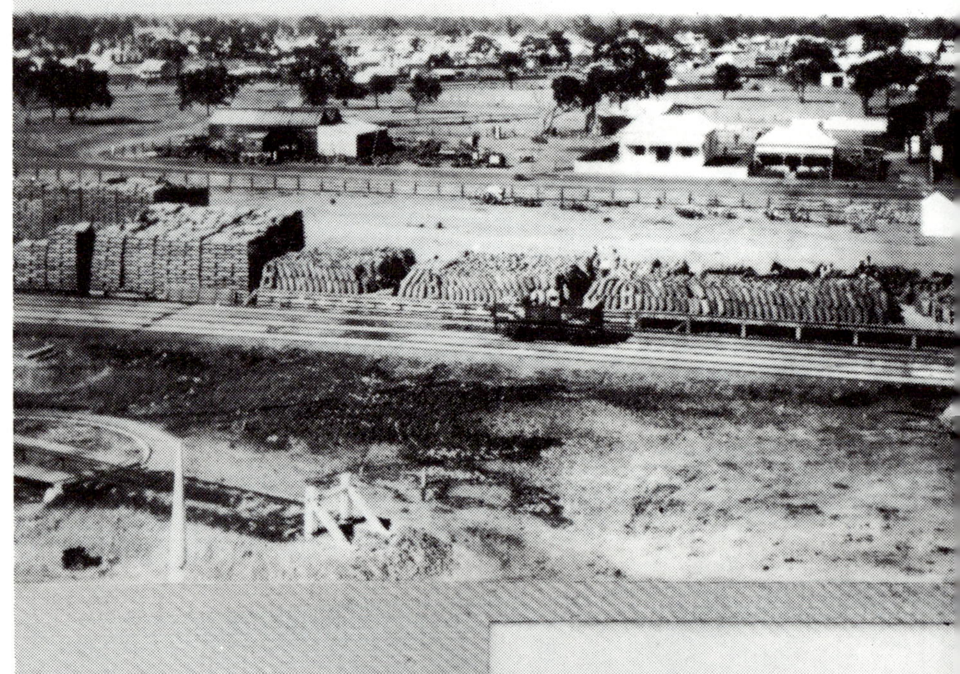

····|··WARRACKNA

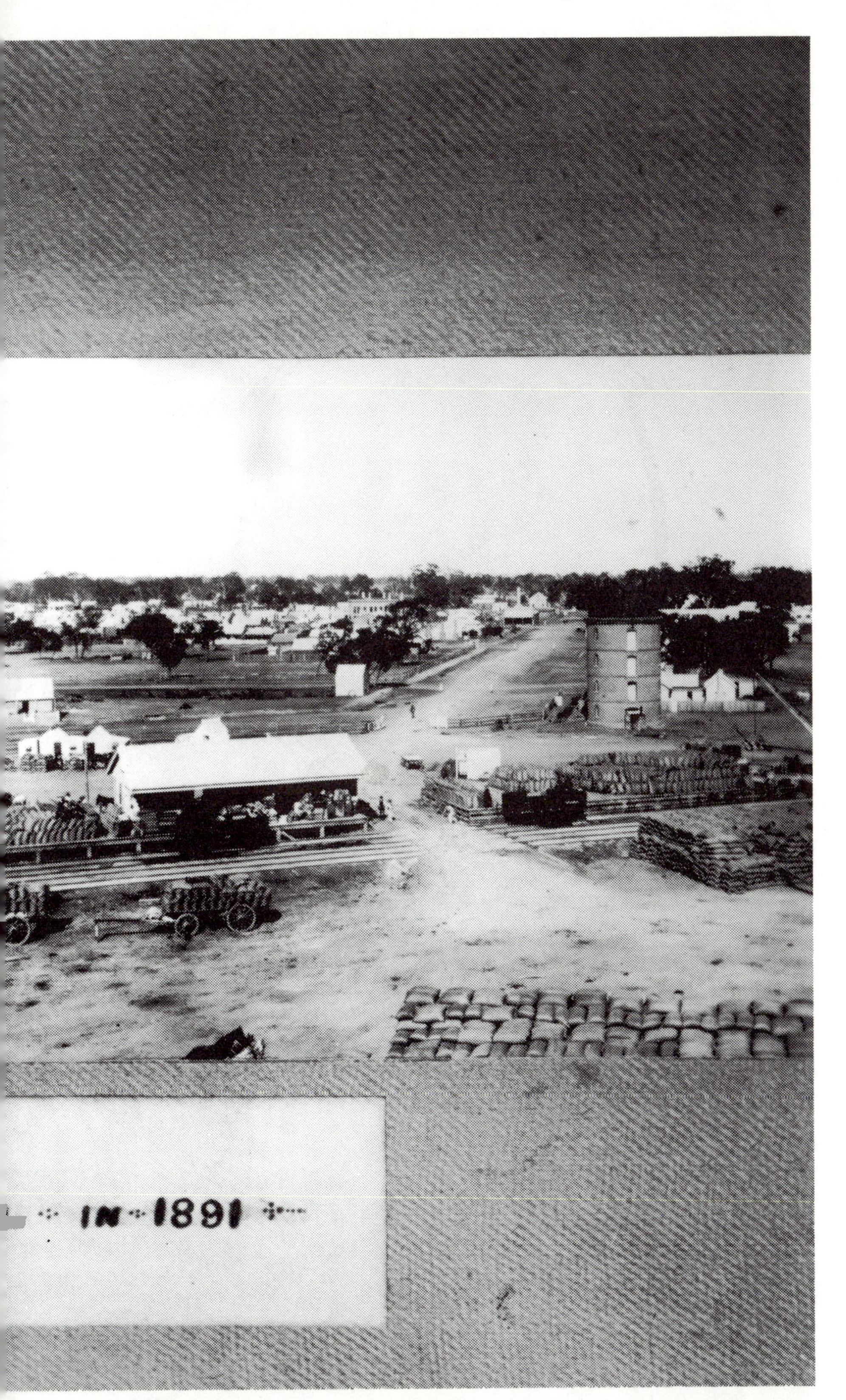
IN 1891

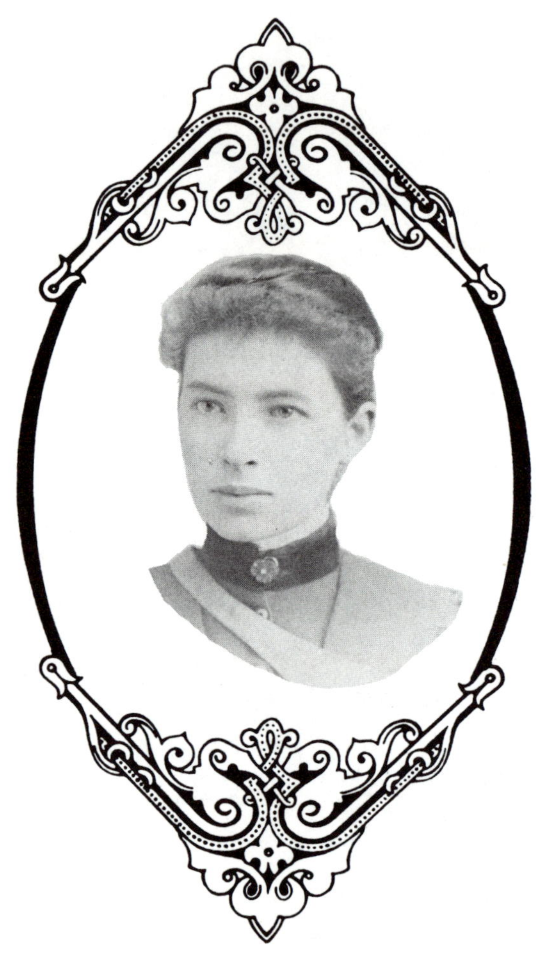

Octavia Grace Ritchie

Dear Grace,

A Romance of History

Margaret Gillett

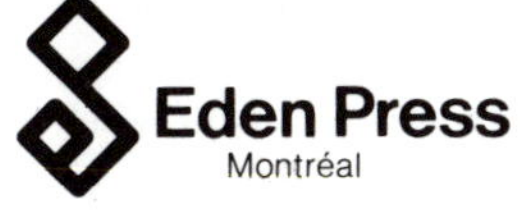

Eden Press
Montréal

DEAR GRACE
A Romance of History
Margaret Gillett

The author gratefully acknowledges research grants from the Social Sciences and Humanities Research Council, Canada, and the Faculty of Graduate Studies and Research, McGill University, Montreal.

ISBN: 0–920792–58–8

Cover illustration: James Watling
Cover design: EDDESIGN
Page design: Evelyne Hertel
Photo credit: page 92, Notman Archives, McCord Museum, McGill University

Printed in Canada at Metropole Litho Inc.
Dépôt légal — troisième trimestre 1986
Bibliothèque nationale du Québec

Eden Press
4626 St. Catherine Street W.
Montreal, Quebec, H3Z 1S3
Canada

Canadian Cataloguing in Publication Data

Little, William C. (William Clow), 1860–1911
    Dear Grace

1. Little, William C. (William Clow), 1860–1911—Correspondence.
2. Ritchie, Grace, 1868–1948-Correspondence.
3. Physicians—Australia—Correspondence. 4. Women physicians—Quebec (Province)—Correspondence. I. Ritchie, Grace 1868–1948 II. Gillett, Margaret, 1930- III. Title.

R674.L48A4 1986   610'.92'4   C86–090183–1

*Dedicated to the memory
of
Isobel L. Wright, M.D.*

TABLE OF CONTENTS

The Romance of Doing History
or
In Pursuit of Billy Little

The Romance of Doing History
or
In Pursuit of Billy Little

Historiography is a formidable word — intimidating, mysterious or even unknown to the world at large. Many people, if they ever give the matter any attention, probably think that the process of writing history is a solitary business, even a dreary one. Dim visions of lonely scholars in dusty archives might flit across their mental screens. They may see the hapless historians accompanied only by ponderous tomes and complicated legal documents, they may see them involved in the painstaking checking and cross-checking of data, laboriously compiling statistics, discerning trends, digging through the overwhelming miscellaneous detritus of years gone by that is known as primary material. All of these seem inevitable parts of the researchers' tasks, which anchor them in gloomy interiors, chain them to library shelves, and bar them from human contact, sunlight and excitement. Perhaps most people do not think of historians and their work in terms like these but, if they do, they are wrong.

As historians know, historical research can be as full of excitement as any other quest, the writing of history as intriguing as the composing of any detective story. Historians may unravel mysteries great and small, have surprise encounters with coincidences, garner great satisfaction from the gathering of scattered clues, and leap imaginatively over dead ends. Even those with the most ascetic of scholarly hearts must feel them beat a little faster as knowledge takes shape and understanding is formed, when unspectacular fragments begin to settle into bright kaleidoscopic patterns of knowledge. Nor are historians necessarily solitary. They may work in teams, or their work may involve many others apart from colleagues — family, friends, even strangers. Historians can build a network of people who, willy-nilly, become fascinated by the researchers' subject.

The letters of William C. Little to Grace Ritchie have provided me with an unexpected but very real opportunity to sample the pleasures of historical discovery. Theirs is a story of an old romance, and the story of their exegesis is a romance in itself.

○ ○ ○

Several years ago, I was engaged in research and writing about the history of women at McGill University in Montreal, Canada. This took me back to the nineteenth century and to the struggles and triumphs of the women who dearly wanted the privilege of higher education. I found myself caught up in the eternal arguments about Woman's "proper" sphere; her "God-given" domestic role, her fundamental unsuitability for intellectual pursuits, and the likelihood of the educated woman being barren or bearing deformed offspring, versus the concept of Woman as a full-fledged human being with intelligence, ambition, and creative abilities, whose achievements were limited only by circumscribed social opportunities and economic dependence. It took a good deal of courage and determination on the part of young women of the Victorian tradition to gain admittance to the colleges and universities in Europe, North America and Australasia. As it turned out, many young women had those necessary qualities. Fortunately, they also had help from sympathetic people in high places (including men) so that they were ultimately successful against prejudice and tradition on the one hand, shyness and embarrassment on the other.

In the process of reconstructing this drama as it had unfolded at McGill, I tried to get as close as possible to those enterprising pioneers. None of the original members of the first class of women admitted to McGill (the class of 1888) was still alive, but their sons and daughters were. What is more, many mementos of their lives as students still remained, just waiting for someone to piece together.

One of the leading women in the original class in the Faculty of Arts was Octavia Grace Ritchie. She was a remarkable woman in many ways, not the least of which was that she never seemed to throw anything away. This habit of keeping drafts of documents, postcards, photographs, and all manner of memorabilia may have coincided with her awareness of being part of a significant historical development, the acceptance of women into higher education. Whether or not she was aware of her historic importance, she left a great deal of primary material that her daughter, Mrs. Esther Cushing, generously gave to me. Later on, when Mrs. Cushing was clearing out the proverbial attic in her mother's summer home in Quebec's Eastern Townships region, she came across a bundle of personal letters written to her mother almost a century ago. As Esther Cushing discovered by glancing through them, these letters had nothing to do with McGill. They seemed to be just part of her mother's accumulated paper avalanche. She tossed a couple into the fire. Then, happily, she reconsidered, reflecting that even though they had nothing to do with McGill, I still might be interested in seeing these letters since most of them came from Australia, and so did I. So Grace Ritchie's daughter offered the letters to me and I eagerly accepted. But somehow they got lost. They were missing for months until, at last, a rather puzzled relative of Mrs. Cushing's asked her why on earth she had sent her a bundle of old letters. Some mistake, surely. The confusion was soon sorted out and the letters of William C. Little, written between 1889 and 1894 to Grace Ritchie, finally fell into my hands.

Although I was extremely interested, the pressures of other work kept me from doing much about these letters for some time. When I was able to count them, sort them into chronological order, read them, make copies, and have a rough draft typed, I had what I thought to be a lively fragment of social history, plus one photograph, three newspaper clippings, one pressed flower, and three eucalyptus gum leaves. Of the twenty-seven letters, the first was written from Edinburgh, Scotland, while the last, and indeed most of them, came from Warracknabeal, a small town in the Australian state of Victoria. There was a large gap for the year 1892. Perhaps those were the ones burned by Esther Cushing, or maybe Grace Ritchie herself had destroyed them for some reason, or perhaps she just never kept them because she was travelling in Europe around that time. We shall probably never know.

What remained, however, seemed to have a certain coherence. The letters were all written by a young Canadian physician to a compatriot in Montreal who was herself in the process of becoming a doctor. In the first letter the writer, who had just acquired post-graduate qualifications, self-mockingly introduced himself in his new guise to his old friend; in the last letter, he rode off into the sunset to shoot kangaroo. In between was a correspondence that revealed a great deal about two young people of the last century, their emotions, their values and their activities. There were also glimpses of life in the Australian bush, comparisons between the Canadian and the Australian ways of doing things, as well as information about medical procedures, details of prescriptions recommended and fees charged a hundred years ago. This might not be earth-shaking stuff, but it was genuinely interesting at the human level and provided a special inside view of some medical history. So it seemed to me that the letters of William Little to Grace Ritchie were of historic value and should be published.

How does one go about doing that? What is the next step? Obviously, no publisher would want to reproduce a random collection of old letters by some totally unknown person. The historian's task here is to find out more about the writer and the recipient, and to provide some socio-historical background so as to place the principals in context. For Grace Ritchie it would be relatively easy. Her daughter and other people who knew her were still alive so that the testimony of these informants, plus her own papers, which I had also been given, would form a strong primary base. Further, because I already knew something about her and her career, I had a fair idea of where to start looking for other and secondary sources, such as in the records of the National Council of Women and Catherine L. Cleverdon's *The Woman Suffrage Movement in Canada* (1950). Finding William C. Little was *une autre histoire*. Mrs. Cushing did not know anything about him other than that he had been an old beau of her mother's. Over the years she had heard her mother speak of "Billy Little" but she could not recall any details. Clearly, the first question to be answered was "Who was Billy Little?"

To begin with, there was sketchy internal evidence from the letters themselves. Although I had never heard of Dr. William C. Little before, I knew from what he wrote that he was born in the region of Barrie, Ontario, on what he called "a crazy day" in 1860. I knew his father was a farmer who later sold the farm and moved to Toronto. I knew he had at least one brother (Jim) and at least four sisters (Maggie, Susie, Lizzie, and Bella). I knew the weights of his sisters (113, 134, 152, and *162*). I did not know (or much care) which one weighed what. I knew he had two cousins, both called Dr. Cross, and that one of them lived in Australia. I knew that he had obtained his M.D. degree at Queen's University in Kingston, Ontario, and guessed that it was there that he met Grace Ritchie. I knew he intended to return to North America in time for the Chicago Exhibition of 1893. Although I could see that he failed to keep that date, I did not know whether he did go home eventually, whether he married, whether he left a family on either side of the Pacific, or where and when he died. For sure I did not know a great deal, but I liked the personality that emerged from between the lines of his letters and I wanted to know more about him.

It seemed to me rather unlikely that William C. Little had made any great medical discoveries or even that he was particularly distinguished. It was probable that he was an ordinary medical person practising in un-exceptional, if unexpected, surroundings. I saw him as Everyman rather than Great Man. If I wanted to know more about him, it was obvious that I would have to spend a considerable amount of time, effort and money in the pursuit. A usual step for any Canadian academic to take at this juncture is to apply for a research grant. That is precisely what I did, requesting funds from the Social Sciences and Humanities Research Council (SSHRC) in order to investigate William C. Little's family background, education and career, and to travel to Australia to explore the record there. I filled out the appropriate forms, met the required deadline and awaited my fate.

In due course the response arrived. It contained a decision and copies of the four reviews of my proposal on which that decision was based. The reviews were, of course, anonymous, but it was clear that three were from people in Canada, the fourth from someone in Australia. Reviews A,C, and D were very positive. The reviewers made agreeable judgments on the project itself and on the competence of the applicant. One (obviously, from the comments, the Australian) was particularly enthusiastic, noting that no similar body of first-hand materials dealing with local medical practice in nineteenth-century Victoria was known to exist, expecting that my work would make a useful contribution to social history by making these unique letters generally accessible. Then there was Reviewer B. Reviewer B was lukewarm. Reviewer B did not dismiss the project or the researcher out of hand, but opined that the whole value of the enterprise depended on the importance of the author of the letters and, since no one had ever heard of William C. Little, it was unlikely that he was of particular significance. Furthermore, Reviewer B doubted whether I would ever be able to discover any information about him.

That gloomy report might have been enough to doom my chance of a grant. Yet in spite of it, the reply of the SSHRC was positive. The grant was not as generous as I had hoped, but it gave me a start. With what might be considered typical Canadian caution, it awarded a small amount of money to cover some clerical expenses and some travel costs in Canada, but nothing for Australia. I personally thought that a visit to Warracknabeal would be crucial to discovering the answer to the question "Who was Billy Little?" but it could wait a while, and I was glad of any encouragement. However, I was determined to succeed, if only to show Reviewer B how wrong he or she was. That really energized my pursuit of Billy Little.

○ ○ ○

The trouble with "Little" is that it is a very common name. There must be thousands of Littles in Canada and in Australia. Luckily, I had some parameters for my quest, so one of the first things I did was to seek out colleagues interested in the history of medicine. These included Dr. Edward Bensley, a former Dean of Medicine at McGill, and Ms. Marilyn Fransiszyn, one of McGill's superbly competent and obliging reference librarians. Both seemed intrigued by my Little project and wished me well. Dr. Bensley suggested I contact certain medical organizations in Ontario and Scotland to trace Dr. Little's registration as a physician, and he provided names and addresses. Ms. Fransiszyn offered to scan the obituary columns of medical journals to try to establish the date of William C. Little's death. I really had no idea when that might have occurred. It was conceivable that he had died soon after writing the last letter. He had not been well then. In fact, he had been on sick leave. So perhaps he had died in 1894 and that was why the letters had stopped — or perhaps not. Of course, I also wanted to know the exact date of his birth and expected that the official records from his birthplace would quickly help me pin down the "crazy day" on which W.C.L. said he was born. Therefore, I wrote to the town clerks of the city of Barrie and the township of Innisfil, making a similar inquiry to the registrar general for the province of Ontario. I guessed at first that the "crazy day" might be April 1, but then I realized that 1860 was a leap year, so maybe February 29 was William Little's birthday, or maybe the day was just "crazy" because something like a howling snow storm happened on it. Who knows?

While I was waiting for some results from these inquiries, I began to look for some more of the substance of the events between W.C.L.'s birth and his death. So I went to the National Archives and Public Library in Ottawa, thinking I would start with the old Barrie and district newspapers. These could be a very fruitful source and I envisioned a local "rag" that carried an exotic story of a Barrie boy making good in the wilds of the remote Antipodes. I also thought it at least possible that "my" William C. Little might appear in one of the multitude of biographical directories published in Canada in the nineteenth and early twentieth centuries, or even in their Australian equivalents. Alas! the files of Barrie newspapers were virtually non-existent in the Canadian National Archives — so no luck there. However, biographical directories abounded. I went systematically through shelf after shelf of them, works such as *Cyclopaedia of Canadian Biography* (1886, 1888, 1919), *Canadian Men and Women of the Time* (1898 and 1912), *National Encyclopedia of Canadian Biography* (1935), *Canadian Who Was Who* (1875–1937), and twenty more, as well as the Ontario *Gazetteer and Directory* (1869–) and *Lovell's Business and Professional Directory* (1882–). The half-dozen Australian biographical directories in the Canadian National Library were no help either. Sure enough, most of them had listings under "Little," but not "my" family.

At the end of a very long morning, the scent warmed a little. There in Ottawa, I found a xeroxed index of a microfilmed scrapbook of biographical information compiled by the Metropolitan Toronto Central Libary. It referred to a Dr. Alfred Thomas Little of Barrie. Much heartened, I hastened to the microfilm section and found the entry. It was an obituary dated either 1937 or 1938 (the date was impossible to decipher) disclosing that Dr. Alfred Thomas Little had been born in Allandale in Innisfil Township, had lived on Maple Street in Barrie, been Barrie Health Officer, and had had two sons. One of these sons was a postal officer in Toronto, the other was Dr. William C. Little, who was associated with his father in medical practice in Barrie. Surely there must be a connection! Same name, same town, same profession. Obviously not my subject, but perhaps a nephew, perhaps named for "my" William C. And in 1982, he was possibly still alive. The most recent (1980) Simcoe County directory confirmed this. There was a Dr. William C. Little practising on Maple Street, Barrie. The current (1982) telephone directory denied it. Again, lots of Littles, but only Mrs. W.C. Little on Peel (not Maple). I feared I was just a bit too late. I reasoned that the doctor must have died and his widow moved. It seemed rather unlikely that she would know much about a possible relative of her husband's who might have died in Australia as long ago as 1894, but it was worth a try.

As soon as I returned to Montreal, I wrote to Mrs. Little explaining my quest and indicating that I would telephone in a few days, to allow time for the letter to reach her and for her to think about the matter. To my surprise, when I phoned an elderly male voice answered and the speaker acknowledged being Dr. William C. Little. He said he had written to me, that he was not feeling well, and that was the end of the conversation. When the eagerly anticipated letter arrived it said:

December 1, 1982

My wife read your letter of the 23 inst. to me.

There has been no Dr. William C. Little born in Barrie. I am Dr. William C. Little and I was born in Churchill a few miles south of Barrie in 1895. My father, Dr. Alfred T. Little, was born near Barrie in 1863. His father, William C. Little was a farmer on the outskirts of Barrie and was born in Glos. England and came to Canada approximately 1840. This is all the information I can give you. My father graduated from Trinity Medical School, Toronto, in 1886.

Yours sincerely

William C. Little, M.D.

There! I had it from himself. There was no other Dr. William C. Little of Barrie. Wrong man. Wrong family. Back to square one.

I was also getting nowhere with the "crazy day" inquiries. Official records were not kept as far back as 1860, or so wrote the deputy city clerk of Barrie on impressive city hall stationary. Even though I filled out forms for the registrar general, sent money and swore that my intentions were honourable, had several exchanges by mail and a long, long-distance telephone conversation, it all came to naught. A consultation of the 1861 manuscript census for Canada West (as Ontario was then called) revealed only sketchy data. While the 1871 census had more family details, on the matter of births it indicated simply that William, son of Robert and Susan Cross Little, was then eleven years old — but I already knew that.

Still, the trail was not yet stone dead. Marilyn Fransiszyn had checked, in the Osler History of Medicine Library, twenty-three medical directories, Canadian, British and American, without success. Her diligence was rewarded to a minor degree when she found our Dr. William C. Little listed under "Barrie, Ontario," in the 1890 edition of *The Doctor in Canada* and again in the *Ontario Medical Register* for 1937, where he appeared under "Deceased Members": "1889– Little, W.C."

Dead in 1889! That would have made him only twenty-nine, and I knew he was still writing letters in 1894. The scanty entry must have referred to the date of his registration, not of his death. An inquiry to the Ontario College of Physicians and Surgeons revealed that they had a listing for him and indicated that he had died in 1923. However, Marilyn continued the search, and the scrutiny of some journals recently returned from the bindery, together with the acquisition of a complete index of the obituaries in the *Canadian Medical Association Journal (CMAJ)*, gave us our first real lead. An entry in the obituary section of the *CMAJ* (Vol. 1, 1911) was almost as terse as the earlier one we had found, but it was more convincing:

> A cable message announces the death of Dr. W.C. Little,
> formerly of Toronto, and at the time of his death practising
> at Warracknabeal, Australia. Dr. Little was a graduate in
> medicine of Queen's University. (p. 1221)

There could be no doubt that this was the right Dr. Little. He had died at fifty-one. That now seemed clearly established, but I still did not know the precise date of his death, only that it had occurred in Australia. It now seemed likely that he had never returned home, but had spent his whole career "down under." It seemed that nothing much would come from the search in Canada. More than ever, I wanted to seek out Billy Little in Australia.

The solution to this problem was remarkably simple. if expensive. Since I was fortunate in having family and friends in Australia and Christmas was approaching, I phoned my sister Mrs. Betty Plaskitt, in Sydney, wondering whether she would care to have a house guest for part of the Christmas vacation. She kindly said she would. I managed to arrange for a slightly extended vacation period and, at quite short notice, made my airline bookings. The fare was high, of course, and the routing horrible. I had to spend endless hours in both directions in the Chicago and Los Angeles airports, and what seemed like days in the air. But I was delighted to be going home for Christmas and excited that my quest was gathering momentum. Either Reviewer B or I would be proved right.

○　○　○

Before I left Montreal, I wrote two very important letters to Australia. The first was to Diana Dyason, Reader in the History and Philosophy of Science at the University of Melbourne. I had learned through the international scholarly network that she was conducting an historical study of the medical profession in Victoria. In my letter to her I outlined my own project, asked if I might visit her in Melbourne, and wondered if she had any suggestions or advice to offer. Her response was prompt and enthusiastic. Among other things, she alerted me to the fact that there were three Warracknabeal newspapers published in the nineteenth century and that they were on file in the La Trobe Library in Melbourne. This was a great help and saved much precious time. I felt confident that somewhere in the pages of the *Warracknabeal Herald,* the *Northern Argus* or the *Warracknabeal and NorthWest Advertiser* I would find news of Dr. Little. The clippings enclosed with his letters to Grace Ritchie indicated as much. They were undated, but I felt I would be able to track them down and find others perhaps more telling than, for example, the one enclosed with a letter from 1890 that read:

> Dr. Little, assisted by Dr. Young, performed a successful operation at the Horsham hospital on Sunday. It was a case of empyema — a large amount of pus having collected in a cavity in the chest, and fully a gallon of liquid was drawn out. The patient, a Chinaman named Charles Ah Wong, is progressing favourably.

With any luck at all, I should be able to discover more of Dr. Little's professional and social activities from these local papers.

The second letter to Australia was much more of a shot in the dark. I addressed it, "for want of better knowledge," simply to "The Mayor, Warracknabeal, Victoria, Australia." I was not sure that Warracknabeal had a mayor. (The little Australian town in which I grew up did not.) Atlases, geography books and the Australian High Commission in Ottawa did not have a great deal to say about Warracknabeal. I gathered, however, that it was a town of about three thousand people in the north-west part of the state, off the main route between Melbourne and Adelaide, on the fringe of the Mallee scrub country, and a centre for sheep and wheat farming. Although in my day, Australian country towns were not noted for their concern for history, and though Dr. Little had been dead for seventy years, there ought to be some official records somewhere of someone who must have been an important member of the community. I must admit that I thought I would probably get more information from the newspapers, hospital records and people's memories than I would through municipal sources, but a hypothetical mayor was a place to start. Town records could show property ownership, marital status, whether there were any descendants, and so on. I indicated in my letter that I planned to visit Warracknabeal, and that I would welcome any help that might be offered. In case it might facilitate communications, I gave my sister's address and phone number in Sydney as a contact point. I mailed this letter with no great expectations, and probably arrived in Australia on about the same day it did.

So it turned out that, thanks to Billy Little, I spent Christmas in Australia in 30-degree weather with wonderful summer food and frivolities, enjoying happily nostalgic visits to family and old school friends.

What is more, the telephone rang. It was not the mayor of Warracknabeal. It was the unofficial mayor. His name was Doug McColl, he was a pharmacist and, incredibly, president of the Warracknabeal Historical Society. In my wildest dreams I had never imagined the existence of such an organization. Doug McColl was just as excited about the whole project as I was. He knew a lot about my Dr. Little. By the strangest coincidence, there was an item on him in the current issue of *Warunda Review,* the Society's quarterly newsletter. An additional item was slated for the next issue. Doug knew where Dr. Little was buried and had a biographical statement about him from *The Cyclopedia of Victoria* (1905, pp. 252-53), and knew where he had lived in Warracknabeal. He had already explored the shire records and believed that Dr. Little had never married and had left no descendants in the town. Mr. McColl was looking forward to my visit and found the timing amazingly provident. Clearly, my next task was to get there.

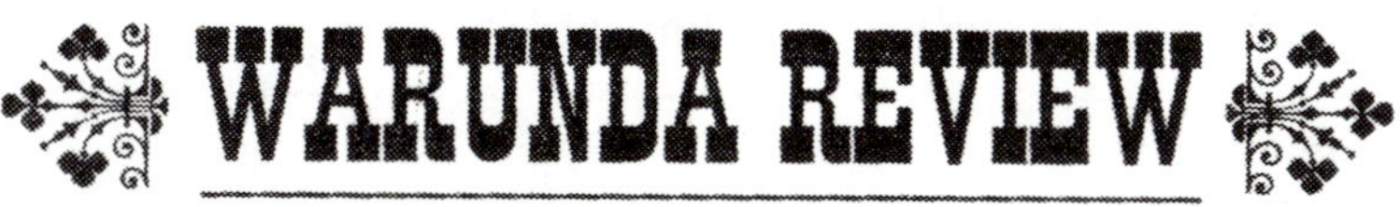

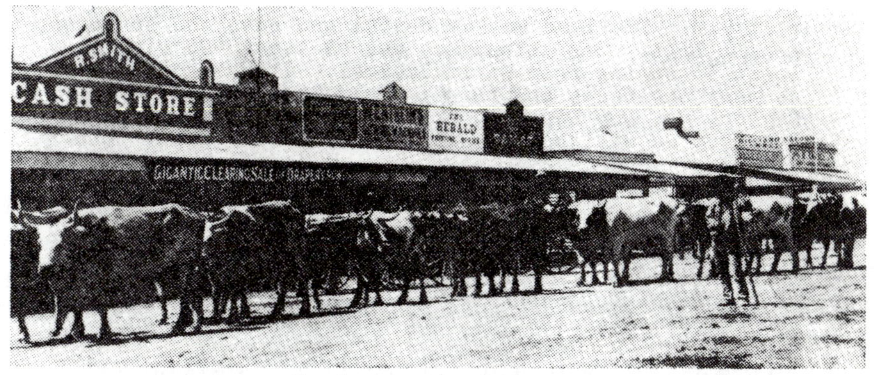

View of Scott Street, Warracknabeal, 1894

The Warracknabeal Historical Society's Quarterly

For someone who had flown thousands of miles across continent and ocean to reach Sydney, getting from that city to a town in the next state should have been no problem at all. Start by going to Melbourne and take it from there. But the Christmas holidays, which coincide with the long summer vacation for schools and everybody else in Australia, plus the hot weather, made transportation difficult. Added to that, there simply seemed no way to get to Warracknabeal — at least no direct way. Once-existent plane, train and bus services seemed to be no more. The most convenient way, then, would be by car, though a very long drive over uncertain conditions and on the "wrong" side of the road did not have a great deal of appeal for me. Luckily, a very happy solution to this dilemma soon presented itself — one I like to think of as "typically Australian" and one that illustrates how the historical research process can involve people. My sister Betty had by now heard a great deal about my quest for Billy Little and she spoke of it to her friends. Indeed, it did make a fine conversation piece. Thus it came to the ears of Joan Utber of Melbourne, who was visiting *her* sister (*my* sister's friend) in Sydney. Joan, whom I had never met, was intrigued by my odyssey as well as curious about the fate of the Canadian migrant in the Australian bush. She not only offered to drive me from Melbourne to Warracknabeal, but also insisted that I stay with her in Melbourne while I was exploring the Warracknabeal papers in the La Trobe Library. Her kind hospitality helped make the next phase both simple and pleasant.

○   ○   ○

On my first morning in Melbourne I went to the office of the Registrar of Births, Deaths and Marriages. I was hoping to obtain a copy of William C. Little's death certificate. I filled in a form, stated my purpose as scholarly research, claimed no connection of kin, confessed to not knowing the exact date of death (except for the year), gave my sister's address in Sydney, paid a little money, and expected the certificate to be mailed in a few days. It was.

The next stop was the La Trobe Library, where the old Warracknabeal newspapers proved to be seductive — not so much the ones on microfilm, but the real ones, which were presented to me in large oblong packages wrapped in voluminous amounts of brittle brown paper and tied with equally generous quantities of shaggy string. They were the genuine old-fashioned, full-sized newspapers, neatly folded in three. To scan them on the flat tables of the reading room of the La Trobe I found it necessary to stand, both so that I could see and so that the unwieldy, fragile newsprint would not tear as I turned the pages. And what pages they were. Those sometimes-smudged black and white sheets were filled with all the colour of a vigorous nineteenth-century community. They contained everything from personal notices to advertisements for miracle patent medicines to a special section announcing the arrival of Wirth's circus; reports of the activities of the local Shire Council and the Vermin Board; gossip parading as social news, school exam results, tennis, horse-racing and cricket scores, prices of wheat, lamb, hogget and mutton; lurid accounts of crimes committed both near and far, reports of world events along with commentary on them, dissertations on droughts, romantic poetry, narrative ballads, serialized novels, and words of inspiration. It was all there.

Because my quarry had arrived in Australia in 1889, I started with the *Warracknabeal Herald* for that year and soon found that I had to exercise great discipline to make myself stay on my own engrossing topic. Items such as the editorial on ''The General Election'' (February 28, 1889) intruded upon my attention. In that piece the writer inveighed against current ''fads'' that had ''found godfathers lately''; ''among such questions we may cite that of women's suffrage, a thing no woman cares a straw about, and no man would think of forcing on womankind. . . .'' Nor could the headline ''A Noted American Female Spy'' (April 4, 1889) be passed over. Under the dateline ''From the Indian Frontier'' was an extraordinary story of a woman who had spied for the South and who was eventually shot. Even advertisements were alluring, especially the long, fantastic puffery of Dr. Frederick Homan, who claimed to be a legally qualified and registered medical practitioner. In that era, before the regulation of professional advertising, Homan offered his "world-renowned services" to:

> Young, middle-aged and elderly men suffering from the results of early follies, transgressions, prostration, loss of energy, love of solitude and moping alone, loss of memory and giddiness, lassitude, no refreshment after sleep, varicose veins, timidity, involuntary blushing, self-distrust, excess bladder difficulties, whitish or dark ropey sediment in the water, accompanied by slight burning or smarting sensation, headaches, drowsiness during the day, circles around the eyes, irregularity of the bowels, specks before the eyes, discontentedness, weakness, pains in the back, liver and kidney complaints, dreams, buzzing noises in the ears and head, pimples, a fear that something is going to happen, weak stomach, yellow and bloodstained eyes, impure blood, hasty uncontrollable temper, hacking cough, who cannot honourably marry, palpitations of the heart, general weakness, and all other symptoms which lead to misery, insanity and death.

Men who had any of the problems mentioned were urged to lose no time in consulting Dr. Homan, who had "cured thousands of these treacherous phantoms, restoring the patient to health and manhood" (April 4, 1889).

I also found myself sympathizing with the Rev. W.H. Evans, who complained (December 5, 1889) that his sermons were frequently interrupted by "yahoos" at the church door; with the local lamplighter who had, for the second time, to replace all his lamps because of "roisterers" who appeared to "know no law but their own sweet will"; with the residents who objected when their gardens were invaded and damaged by their neighbour's pigs (July 18, 1889); and with the girl who "while engaged in cleaning out the ladies' waiting room at St. Kilda railway station . . . discovered the dead body of a newly born fully developed female child in a cupboard under the washbasin" (January 16. 1890). All this fascinating material, the stuff of life, was not simply an unwarranted diversion (so I rationalized for myself), it helped paint a picture of the world into which my Dr. William C. Little was about to plunge.

I had also thought there might just possibly be some discussion about the status of medical services in Warracknabeal, the need for new doctors, or some indication of his impending arrival. However, I found nothing until I came to the "Special Advertisement" column on the front page of the January 30, 1890, issue. Here, along with the announcements of another physician, two solicitors, two dentists, one engineer, one architect, one surveyor and one Chinese herbalist, was the following discreet entry:

WILLIAM C. LITTLE, M.D., Ch.M.
Member of the College of Physicians
and Surgeons of Ontario
Licentiate, Royal College of Surgeons,
Edinburgh; and
Fellow of the Obstetrical Society

SURGERY
Phillips Street, Warracknabeal

This discovery had a curiously familiar look and it proved to be one of the undated clippings William Little had sent Grace Ritchie. On the back of that copy he had written: "Terrible ad., isn't it? New Drs. always put in their qualifications. It is not done for show." Such a modest comment presents a marked contrast to the bombastic claims of the good doctor Homan who promised to cure everything. Dr. Little's entry to Warracknabeal seemed to be very low key, but his notice was followed by a brief comment on page two that said simply:

> It will be seen by the advertisement elsewhere that W.C. Little, M.D., Ch.M. has started the practice of his profession in Warracknabeal. We understand that he has secured a lease of the residence of Mr. G. Simpson in Phillips St., where he may be consulted.

The morning of my second day in the La Trobe produced some items about Dr. Little's medical cases similar to the one about draining fluid from the Chinaman's lung, about his being appointed to the staff of the hospital in Horsham (a nearby town), about his winning prizes for his horses, and his awarding prizes to lady riders. It was slow going but fairly fruitful. The highlight of the day was lunch at the University of Melbourne with Diana ("Ding") Dyason and two of her colleagues. "Ding" Dyason was engaged in a throughgoing compilation of medical practitioners in the State of Victoria in the nineteenth century. Her computer had William Clow Little and his qualifications duly listed. I believe this was the first time I had seen his second name in full. (The Canadian manuscript census gives only "William.") Ms. Dyason's record also showed that he, like other legitimate physicians, was registered with the Victorian Medical Board. However, he was listed only to 1901. Why 1901? Why not longer? Why not until, 1911, or at least closer to the time of his death?

I returned to the La Trobe realizing that, because of the limited time available, I could not go through every paper looking for miscellaneous items about Dr. Little. Now that I had substantiated his existence and acquired some of the flavour of his time and place, I would have to concentrate on the potentially most interesting periods. The years 1901 and 1911 were good candidates. The latter seemed to be the more straightforward and, since I did not know the exact date of his demise, I began in January. It took some time to reach the issue of Tuesday, October 10, 1911, where I found his obituary.

Dr. W. C. Little

It is with deep regret that we have to announce the death of Dr. William Clow Little, which occurred on Friday October 6, 1911 at the age of 51 years. Deceased had not been in good health for some time. Last week he left for Melbourne to be under the care of Dr. Stirling, but on Friday he died from an acute attack of pneumonia. Deceased was born in Barrie, county Ontario, Canada in 1860, and was the son of Robert Little, J.P. of that town. He was educated at the Collegiate Institute, Barrie, and Queen's University, Ontario. He also attended the Ontario Agricultural College for two years. He went through a course of science and scientific farming and subsequently gained first prize for an essay on "Livestock," given by the Ontario Government. Dr. Little first came to Victoria to act as locum for his cousin, Dr. Cross, who had a practice in the Western district. At the conclusion of his stay there he settled in Warracknabeal where he quickly built up a large practice. For ten years he was surgeon at the local hospital and also medical officer to the Borong Shire Council. For many years deceased conducted a private hospital, which was in charge of Nurse Gaff. His skill as a surgeon was widely known. Outside his professional life he went in largely for live stock and farming, and he was always ready to aid in anything for the advancement of the town and district. Failing health compelled him to take a trip to recuperate and he sailed around the world. He returned to Warracknabeal recently but his health did not improve and he left for the metropolis to undergo medical treatment, where he died as stated. The deceased was long and favorably known in Warracknabeal and the Wimmera generally, and his death caused keen regret. The funeral took place in Melbourne on Saturday.

Since xerox facilities were not readily available, I copied all this out in mandatory pencil — and I did so with a macabre sort of glee. All that information! Some of it new (the private hospital, Nurse Gaff, the trip around the world), some of it inaccurate (his father was not strictly from Barrie), some of it puzzling (his attendance at the Ontario Agricultural College and the prize for the essay on livestock). This was a veritable jackpot, which Joan Utber and I celebrated fittingly that evening.

○   ○   ○

Time was running out. We were off to Warracknabeal on Friday and soon I was to leave Australia. Yet in my examination of *The Northern Argus* for 1901, I could not resist pausing to read a couple of items that touched upon Canada. One noted that the Catholic clergy of Montreal had strongly advised their flocks not to extend any aid to a visiting Home Rule delegation from Ireland (April 30, 1891), another reported that the Canadian Government had requested the release of some sealers captured by Russian war vessels in the Bering Sea (October 1, 1891). These random items suggested that the Warracknabeal papers were keeping their eyes on the world, but it was the affairs of Warracknabeal itself that were of real interest to me. I had to ignore the reporting of the Australian federation of 1901 and stick to Billy Little. I learned that he had cared for various patients in Nurse Gaff's private hospital throughout the year and then, in the issue from December 10, 1901, my attention was grabbed by a dramatic headline: "The Hospital Trouble." There was a scandal at the Warracknabeal District Hospital and Dr. Little was involved.

The report was not very clear. Both the reporter and writers of letters to the editor felt strongly on the matter and seemed to assume that the readers were familiar with the case. Indeed, all of Warracknabeal in 1901 doubtless knew what was going on. I had to try to piece it together. One thing was certain: Dr. Little was out. There seemed to be several issues involved, one having to do with a benefit concert for the hospital, one concerning membership of the hospital board, and one dealing with a particular medical patient. The latter was the clearest to me. It seemed that Dr. Little had refused, for whatever reason, to perform surgery on behalf of Dr. Ross, an absent colleague, without a written request by the hospital committee. Dr. Ross returned to Warracknabeal and performed the operation; Dr. Little did not participate. Why Little acted as he did was not apparent, but letters in the paper seemed to be on his side. One correspondent who called him/herself "Honest Plain Speaking" attacked the self-complacency of the hospital committee and, in calling for an inquiry, implied that there was "a plot to dispense with Dr. Little's services." Another writer was sure that "the loss is on the side of the hospital in losing his services."

My time had run out. The library was closing for the night. My stay in Melbourne was at an end, but many papers remained unread and many questions unanswered. At least I could now guess that Dr. William Little had failed to renew his membership in the Medical Board because he was no longer officially part of the medical bureaucracy and consequently rejected the formal organization. What the real reasons behind the story were, I did not know. Perhaps they would be revealed in Warracknabeal.

The night before Joan Utber and I set off for Warracknabeal we were as excited as children on Christmas Eve. We could hardly sleep. Joan was now thoroughly involved and had had a couple of telephone conversations with Doug McColl to get directions for our route. She, too, was intrigued by the prospect of unearthing this unknown Canadian and fitting together the clues that were beginning to accumulate. She had also been infected by Doug McColl's enthusiasm, so that we were both looking forward to meeting him and his wife, Evelyn. They had made accommodation arrangements for us at a local motel and would be awaiting our arrival.

We left early in the morning and headed north-west, driving through Ballarat, once notable as a gold-mining town, now distinguished for, among other things, its fine public park with its black swans. It was the hottest time of year, and the country was enduring one of the worst droughts on record, yet I was pleased that we were in that part of the state because I had made some associations between "my" William Little and Henry Handel Richardson's Richard Mahony. When I was at school in Australia I had been devoted to *The Fortunes of Richard Mahony*, then considered *the* Australian novel. It is a trilogy dealing with the adventures — really the rise and descent into madness — of an Irish/English doctor in that area of the country in the mid-nineteenth century. The period was just a bit earlier than that of my subject but the rugged, stubborn countryside and the vagaries of the weather that dominated life here remain unchanged even today.

Perhaps Dr. Little's life had not been quite as dramatic as Dr. Mahony's, but the two doctors had many things in common, including an interest in hypnotism. I had read the book again just recently and was struck by the reference to Mahony's attending a lecture on mesmerism. In the letters to Grace Ritchie I had been surprised to find that Dr. Little had used hypnotism as an anaesthetic. (Such a "modern" technique seemed so out of place in the nineteenth-century bush that I was led to check on the development of hypnotism, to discover that Franz Mesmer lived from about 1733 to 1815, so Dr. Little's technique was not so modern after all, but was probably considered unorthodox in Warracknabeal.)

The road to Warracknabeal proved to be well paved and clearly marked, so that Joan and I had neither difficulty getting there nor in contacting the McColls. They were both extremely affable and had a tightly packed agenda prepared for us. Evelyn escorted us to the Warracknabeal Historical Centre, which is run by the Warracknabeal and District Historical Society. Originally designed as a bank, it was a solid old building of red and light-coloured stone and brick, ornately pillared and crenellated. The front section of the main floor is now preserved as a bank of yesteryear and contains hand-written, leather-bound ledgers and other appropriate artifacts, while the areas to the rear and upstairs hold a plethora of domestic and commercial memorabilia (such as apothecary's equipment) attractively presented in context. It gave us, in concentrated form, a sense of the district's past.

Next, we went to visit several elderly people — one in her home, the others in a special section of the District Hospital — all of whom had personal or family stories of Dr. Little to recount. Some of the details of this anecdotal evidence did not fit with what I considered to be established facts — but the tone emanating from these interviews consistently implied that Dr. Little was a hardworking, enterprising, much-respected, and even a loved personage in Warracknabeal. There was also some mention of odd behaviour towards the end of his life.

Then, thanks to the foresight of the McColls and the kindness of the present owner of the house at 11 Phillips Street (who was out of town at the time but had left her keys with our hosts), we were given an inspection tour of the place where William Little had lived and had his practice. Later, as we drove down Jamoineau Street, Doug pointed out a private residence that now stands on the site once occupied by the Little/Gaff hospital. "In Dr. Little's day," Doug said, "it had a funny name. He called it Massawippi." "Oh!" I said, "Massawippi!" and must have smiled, because that is exactly the reaction of every Canadian to whom I have mentioned this as they instantly recognize the name of a lake in Quebec's Eastern Townships region. Finally, we visited the offices of the *Warracknabeal Herald*, which still publishes once a week. The current issue had just come out and we were astounded (though, given Doug's efficiency we should not have been) to see a large headline at the bottom of page one: "Canadian researcher in Warrack today." The article briefly sketched my mission and asked anyone who had any information about Dr. William C. Little to get in touch with Mr. Doug McColl, president of the Warracknabeal Historical Society. That invitation was to bear some fruit from people's memories and from their family photograph albums.

That evening after dinner at the McColls' delightful home on the banks of the Yarriambac Creek, there was a chance to discuss with Doug in greater detail the material he had collected on Dr. Little. The first item was the biography from *The Cyclopedia of Victoria*. To my delight, it contained a handsome photograph of Dr. William Clow Little, seated and looking very prosperous. The picture showed a sturdy, dark-haired man in his prime, with a high forehead and clear, penetrating eyes. He sported a luxuriant moustache on his upper lip, a carnation in his buttonhole, and a gold watch-chain across his middle. Without doubt, the biographical entry had been written by the subject himself, or at the very least, he had contributed the information and approved the contents. These were very similar to the substance of the obituary I had discovered and, most likely, its source — thus the source of the puzzling reference to the Ontario Agricultural College and the prize essay. Indeed, there was more here that I found curious. The entry said:

> He was appointed by the Government of Canada to proceed
> to England and take charge of stock purchased at the late
> Queen's farm, Windsor, England, for the Canadian Govern-
> ment, and safely transport them back to Canada. (p.252)

When could Billy Little possibly have done that? By my calculations, he had been twenty-nine when he graduated with his M.D. from Queen's, so that he was probably about twenty-five when he first registered there. Was he already such an expert in livestock that the Government of Canada would have charged him with such an important responsibility as transporting select stock from the royal herd? Something seemed wrong.

Most intriguing of all was the item that had been printed in the *Warunda Review*. I discovered that the reason why an article on William C. Little should suddenly appear in the Historical Society's newsletter was that John Schubert, son of the editor, had happened to come across this material. John Schubert is a teacher who lives in Melbourne and who, through one of his friends, was given access to a privately produced history of a family called Steel. What was published in the *Warunda Review* was an extract of this "Steel Family History," and the connection was that Nurse Jenny Gaff had been Jenny Steel. The section in the family history dealing with Dr. Little had been based on her diaries. All of this was a revelation to me because before I went to Australia, I had no inkling of the existence of Jenny Steel Gaff. There is no hint of her in William Little's letters to Grace Ritchie. How I wanted to get my hands on that history and those diaries! And how I marvelled at the coincidence that had brought all this information to light just as I was making my inquiries.

Since some of the material was a repeat of the cyclopaedia article, what fascinated me most about the *Warunda Review* extract was the perspective. This perspective, of course, was that of Jenny Gaff and, if Grace Ritchie had never heard of her, it seems likely she had never heard of Grace Ritchie. The extract begins:

> One of the earliest cases Jenny took was at Camperdown and while there she met Dr. William Little, a Scotch-Canadian. He was practising at Warracknabeal and he urged Jenny to leave private nursing and come to Warracknabeal to help in the Public Hospital where they were desperate for staff. She went and this marked the beginning of their long association which lasted till his death in 1911.

> Dr. Little fell in love with Jenny and wanted to marry her. She was probably very much against marrying again but she became completely devoted to him eventually . . . .

> . . . Their attachment grew stronger and they finally decided to try and find Jenny's husband, as she was not free to marry if he was still alive, and the Doctor had strong views on marrying a divorced woman. He spent much time and money trying to trace Dan Gaff, Snr. Jenny Gaff had a son called Dan, but apart from learning that he'd gone to America when Jenny left Scotland, Dan had disappeared and nothing more was ever heard of him.

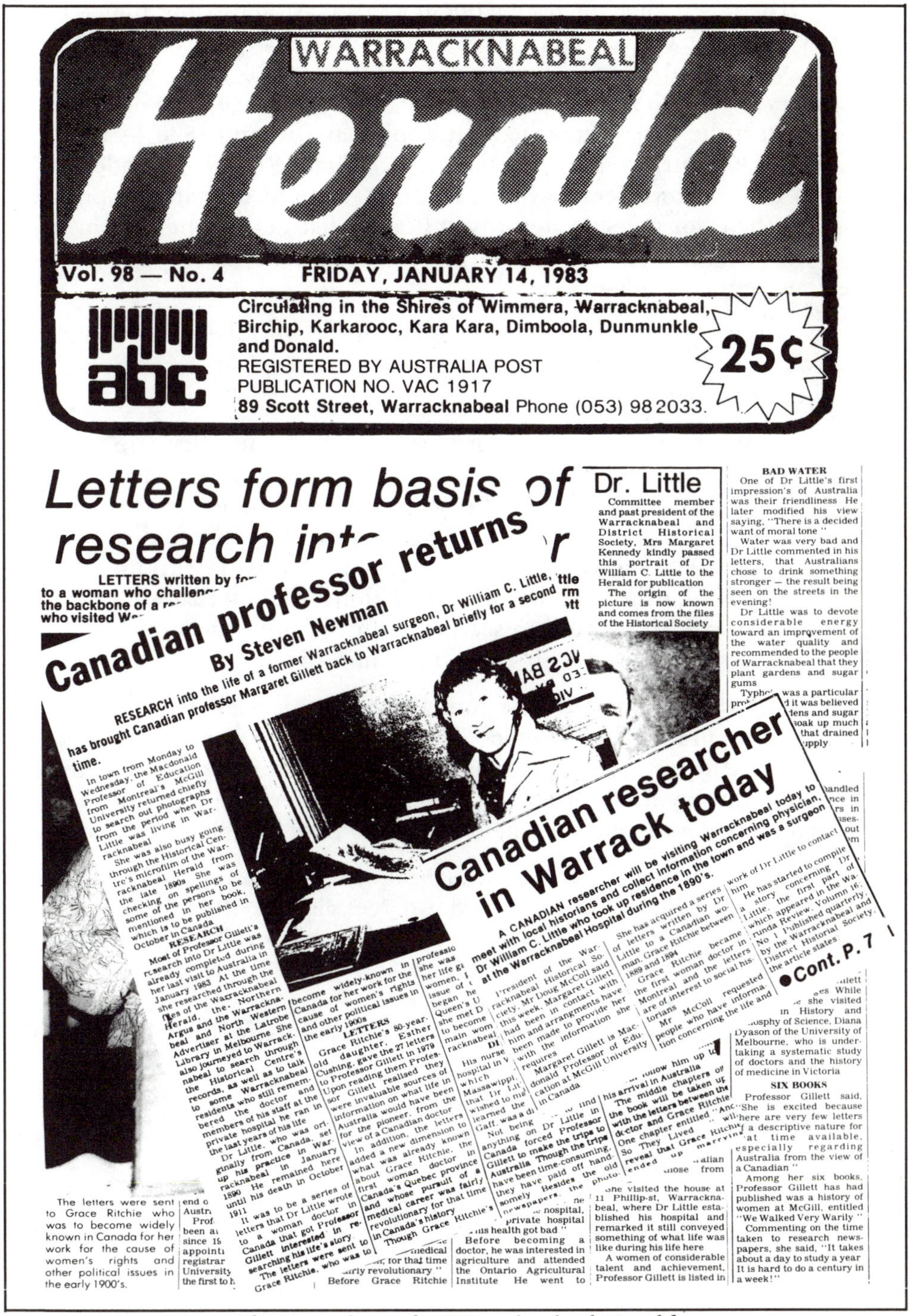

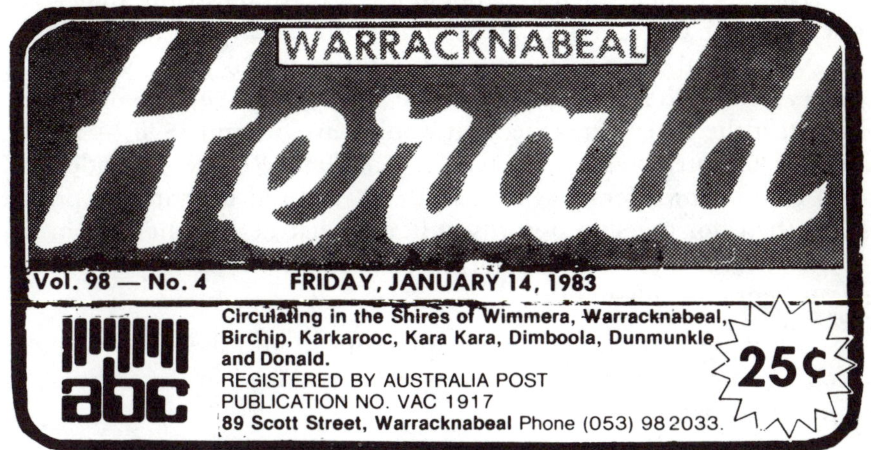

WARRACKNABEAL **Herald**

Vol. 98 — No. 4 FRIDAY, JANUARY 14, 1983

Circulating in the Shires of Wimmera, Warracknabeal, Birchip, Karkarooc, Kara Kara, Dimboola, Dunmunkle and Donald.
REGISTERED BY AUSTRALIA POST
PUBLICATION NO. VAC 1917
89 Scott Street, Warracknabeal Phone (053) 98 2033.

25¢

abc

Letters form basis of research int... r

LETTERS written by fo... to a woman who challen... the backbone of a ... who visited W...

Dr. Little

Committee member and past president of the Warracknabeal and District Historical Society, Mrs Margaret Kennedy kindly passed this portrait of Dr William C. Little to the Herald for publication

The origin of the picture is now known and comes from the files of the Historical Society

BAD WATER

One of Dr Little's first impression's of Australia was their friendliness He later modified his view saying, "There is a decided want of moral tone "

Water was very bad and Dr Little commented in his letters, that Australians chose to drink something stronger — the result being seen on the streets in the evening!

Dr Little was to devote considerable energy toward an improvement of the water quality and recommended to the people of Warracknabeal that they plant gardens and sugar gums

Typho... was a particular pro... it was believed ...dens and sugar ...soak up much ... that drained ...upply

Canadian professor returns

By Steven Newman

RESEARCH into the life of a former Warracknabeal surgeon, Dr William C. Little, has brought Canadian professor Margaret Gillett back to Warracknabeal briefly for a second time.

In town from Monday to Wednesday, the Macdonald Professor of Education from Montreal's McGill University returned chiefly to search out photographs from the period when Dr Little was living in Warracknabeal

She was also busy going through the Historical Centre's microfilm of the Warracknabeal Herald from the late 1890s She was checking on spellings of some of the persons to be mentioned in her book, which is to be published in October in Canada

RESEARCH

Most of Professor Gillett's research into Dr Little was already completed during her last visit to Australia in January 1983 At the time she researched through the files of the Warracknabeal Herald, the Northern Argus and the Warracknabeal and North Western Advertiser at the Latrobe Library in Melbourne She also journeyed to Warracknabeal to search through the Historical Centre's records, as well as to talk to some Warracknabeal residents who still remembered the doctor and members of his staff at the private hospital he ran in the last years of his life

Dr Little, who was originally from Canada, set up his practice in Warracknabeal in January 1890 He remained here until his death in October 1911

It was to be a series of letters that Dr Little wrote to a woman doctor in Canada that got Professor Gillett interested in researching his life's story

The letters were sent to Grace Ritchie, who was to become widely-known in Canada for her work for the cause of women's rights and other political issues in the early 1900s

LETTERS

Grace Ritchie's 80-year-old daughter, Esther Cushing, gave the 27 letters to Professor Gillett in 1979 Upon reading them Professor Gillett realised they were invaluable sources of information on what life in Australia would have been for the pioneer, from the view of a Canadian doctor

In addition, the letters added a new dimension to what was already known about Grace Ritchie, the first woman doctor in Canada's Quebec province and whose pursuit of a medical career was fairly revolutionary for that time in Canada's history

Though Grace Ritchie's ... medical ... for that time ...irly revolutionary "

Before Grace Ritchie

professio... she was ... her life g... women, ... issue of ... began he... Queen's U... she met D... to become ... main wom... racknabeal

D...

His nurse ... hospital in ... which Massawippi, ... that Dr Lit... wished to ma... learned the Gaff, was a d...

Not being ... anything on Dr Little in Canada forced Professor Gillett to make the trips to Australia Though the trips have been time-consuming, they have paid off handsomely Besides the old newspapers, the photo... ... ne ... hospital, ... private hospital ... his health got bad "

Before becoming a doctor, he was interested in agriculture and attended the Ontario Agricultural Institute He went to

The letters were sent to Grace Ritchie who was to become widely known in Canada for her work for the cause of women's rights and other political issues in the early 1900's.

end o... Austr... Prof... been a... since 1... appoint... registrar University the first to h...

Canadian researcher in Warrack today

A CANADIAN researcher will be visiting Warracknabeal today to meet with local historians and collect information concerning physician, Dr William C. Little who took up residence in the town and was a surgeon at the Warracknabeal Hospital during the 1890's.

President of the Warracknabeal Historical Society, Mr Doug McColl said this week, Margaret Gillett had been in contact with him and arrangments have been made to provide her with the information she requires

Margaret Gillett is Macdonald Professor of Education at McGill University in Canada

She has acquired a series of letters written by Dr Little to a Canadian woman, Grace Ritchie between 1889 and 1894

Grace Ritchie became the first woman doctor in Montreal and the letters are of interest to social historians

Mr McColl requested people who have information concerning the life and work of Dr Little to contact him

He has started to compile a story concerning Dr Little, the first part of which appeared in the Warrunda Review, Volumn 16, No 1 Published quarterly by the Warracknabeal and District Historical Society, the article states:

●Cont. P. 7

... follow him up to his arrival in Australia The middle chapters of the book will be taken up with the letters between the doctor and Grace Ritchie One chapter entitled "An... wil... So They Lived ... " will reveal that Grace Ritchie ... marrying ... up ... ended ... ...alian ... those from

She visited the house at 11 Phillip-st, Warracknabeal, where Dr Little established his hospital and remarked it still conveyed something of what life was like during his life here

A women of considerable talent and achievement, Professor Gillett is listed in

...illett ...es While ... she visited ... in History and ...osphy of Science, Diana Dyason of the University of Melbourne, who is undertaking a systematic study of doctors and the history of medicine in Victoria

SIX BOOKS

Professor Gillett said, "She is excited because there are very few letters of a descriptive nature for that time available, especially regarding Australia from the view of a Canadian "

Among her six books, Professor Gillett has had published was a history of women at McGill, entitled "We Walked Very Warily "

Commenting on the time taken to research newspapers, she said, "It takes about a day to study a year It is hard to do a century in a week!"

Clippings from the Warracknabeal Herald

This raised some interesting questions. When did this love affair start? At one point the extract says, "He started a private hospital in Jamoineau Street, Warracknabeal, and Jenny ran it for him for 20 years. When they met, they were both mature people of the same age — 30." No dates were given, but if the latter were true, that would have been in 1890 — that is, while William Little was writing regularly to Grace Ritchie. I wondered if he had really known Jenny as long as that? And did he start the private hospital then, for the shire records indicated that he bought it from her in 1902? There is a caution here for the historian not to accept even seemingly authentic details lightly.

But if the extract raised some questions, it also shed a lot of light. It accounted for the trip around the world mentioned in the obituary in the following manner:

> In March, 1910, William Little took Jenny for her first trip around the world, but he was ill many times during their period away. In her diary she says she was frightened by the thought of being alone in a strange country if he should die. After one of the attacks she said, "The four days of delirium was awful, night and day picking up things for him that were not there.* It's pitiful to see such a fine man in such a terrible state. How I wish I could get him better."

They apparently had an extensive tour and "saw practically everything you could think of in Britain and Europe." They returned to Australia via Canada, where a visit to his parents is mentioned, as well as a stop at Vancouver. Did they also stay in Montreal? If so, did they meet Grace Ritchie? I felt we were on the verge of learning a lot about Billy Little.

Joan Utber and I left Warracknabeal with our heads spinning. There had been a press interview (published two weeks later in the *Warracknabeal Herald*), we had acquired a copy of a book on the history of the town (Susan Priestly, *Warracknabeal: A Wimmera Centenary*, Melbourne: The Jacaranda Press, 1967), and we had been met with tremendous co-operation, intelligent planning, and genuine friendliness. What a successful trip it had been. Nuts to Reviewer B!

o   o   o

---

* The diary actually reads "The four days of delirium was awful, night and day picking up things that were not there."

One of the first things I did when I returned to Montreal was to write to John Schubert in Melbourne. I explained my project, told of the recent visit to Warracknabeal, indicated that I would like to read "The Steel Family" and Jenny Gaff's diaries, which I assumed to be unpublished, and asked for his suggestions about getting them. For a long time there was no reply, even though Joan helped with some local telephone calls from Melbourne. A year passed. Then, greatly to my surprise, I received a very cordial (and slightly apologetic) letter from John Schubert. What is more, he enclosed a xerox copy of "The Steel Family," which proved to be a thirty-three-page typed document. Mr. Schubert explained that he had been in touch with Mrs. Gwen Steel, the author of the family history, and she had assured him that everything concerning Dr. Little that was in Jenny Gaff's diaries was included in the piece that had appeared in the *Warunda Review*. However, she did add one or two further details, as well as comments from two people who had personally known or known of Dr. Little. John Schubert reported that Mrs. Steel said "the diaries were too boring to photocopy." She said they were full of cryptic abbreviations and references to "Mrs. S., Mr. B., etc. without a hint of who the people were." John Schubert was not entirely convinced that I would find the diaries boring — neither was I.

Although he could not deliver the diaries, John Schubert gave me Mrs. Steel's address so that I could write to her myself. When I did so, I asked not for the diaries, with which she understandably seemed unwilling to part, but requested answers to specific questions. These were questions such as: "Did Dr. Little and Nurse Gaff visit Montreal?" "Whom did they see there?" "Was there any trace of Grace Ritchie?" Mrs. Steel then went to a great deal of trouble to examine the "boring" diaries once again. She reported to me that there were no references to Grace Ritchie, but that they did visit Montreal. They stayed at the Windsor Hotel for two nights, and "saw McGill University and all the splendid colleges," before they continued their journey on to Ottawa. She also gave me additional details of the world tour and some of the people they met in Britain and Canada, including the fact that they stayed eight days in Nova Scotia with a "delightful family named Chase who made Jenny feel one of the family." More than that did not seem possible. The rest would have to wait until I had a chance to visit Australia again, when, if Mrs. Steel would permit me, I might examine Nurse Jenny Gaff's diaries for myself.

I must pause here to note how much I appreciated the efforts that both John Schubert and Gwen Steel made on my behalf. John Schubert mentioned in his letter that "as one who has been involved in much family and local historical research, I appreciate the need to ask favours of strangers . . . ." I was very sensitive to the fact that I had asked many favours of strangers and responded to Mr. Schubert in all sincerity that I greatly appreciated the trouble to which he had gone. I told him that "this whole project has been built up by the kindness of people whom I do not really know but who seem to have found it of interest." This is the truth, but I have to confess, not the entire truth. It is not only strangers (like Doug and Evelyn McColl, Joan Utber, the informants in Warracknabeal, archivists, and reference librarians) who have done me favours through this project. Some of those who have helped very significantly were friends I knew well.

Foremost among these was the late Dr. Isobel L. Wright, who lived with me during most of my pursuit of Billy Little. Not only were her interest and support encouraging, but her professional knowledge was invaluable. This was called into play many times as another friend, Miss Muriel Roberts, and I fine-toothcombed our way through Dr. Little's letters to Grace Ritchie. We were trying to produce an exact text. Sometimes we stumbled over indecipherable words, were confounded by medical terms, or puzzled by gnostic abbreviations. Dr. Wright helped us with these and also gave us her opinion of some of Dr. Little's medical procedures — but perhaps professional discretion dictates that this be left unreported! My sister, Betty Plaskitt, who is a pharmacist, also interpreted the prescriptions that Dr. Little passed on to medical student Grace Ritchie; while Dr. Edward Bensley explained some of W.C.L.'s nineteenth-century therapies and their context. Also, Esther Cushing kindly let me interview her several times on the subject of her mother and it was she, of course, who had given me the letters that started the whole thing.

Throughout my investigations, help has come spontaneously. It came, for example, quite unexpectedly as a result of a delightful lunch in the garden of the Art Gallery of Ontario in Toronto with Dr. Elizabeth Rowlinson, Dean of St. Hilda's College, Toronto, and former Associate Dean of Students at McGill. As a conversation piece, I embarked upon my tale of the Billy Little letters, mentioning that he came from the Barrie area. Elizabeth, who has a cottage in that general vicinity, at once volunteered to locate the old Little farm and generally explore the family background. I like to think she thoroughly enjoyed her part in the pursuit of Billy Little. It was a very productive contribution.

In what seemed like no time at all, she had produced from the Ontario Archives a copy of the 1871 manuscript census, Schedule 1 "Nominal Return of the Living," with most of the family of Robert Little (William's father) listed, along with summaries of other schedules showing the number of acres, livestock, and produce of the farm. She also sent xeroxes of two maps of Simcoe County (1871 and 1881). With these, and the information from the *Simcoe Farmers' Directory* for 1890, which located Robert Little, freeholder, at Concession 6, Lot 7, Killyleagh in Innisfil Township, we could determine the exact place where the Little farm had been. Most exciting, she had a copy of the Innisfil Township Centennial (1850-1950) *Historical Review*. This contained brief essays on pioneer families, including "my" Littles. (Coincidentally, the next entry, on another Little family, was contributed by W.C. Little, M.D., presumably the person who had written to me from Barrie.) I had previously obtained a copy of the essay on "my" Littles from the Simcoe County Archives, but had not seen the entire booklet, which was well worth having, especially since Elizabeth read it thoroughly and went to the trouble of cross-indexing random references to Littles or Crosses ("my" William's mother's family).

That was not all. Elizabeth Rowlinson also joined in the search for the "crazy day," William Clow Little's birthday, by making inquiries at the Ontario Archives, the Archives of the Presbyterian Church of Canada, Archives of the United Church of Canada, Simcoe County Archives, Simcoe County Museum, Barrie Library, and the Churchill United Church. All these proved to be dead ends but her inquiries continued undaunted.

The imagination and cheerful energy that went into Elizabeth's investigations comes through in her research notes, for example:

> August 30
>
> Checked 6th Line Cemetery (Presbyterian) — no Littles. Spoke to Mr. Ross Wallace, member of local historical society — no luck, but he suggested I call Mr. Frank Cowan, who is now in his eighties and lived in Innisfil all his life. He remembers his grandfather speaking of the Littles on the 6th Line — "They were a very fine family" — but no details.
>
> Asked at Innisfil Township Office where working papers for *Historical Review* would be — they didn't know. All committee members for the book are now dead.
>
> Went to the house on Robert Little's farm — looks late 19th century (typical Ontario country house of the time — red brick with quite ornate wood trim — now rather shabby). Woman said, "A George Little used to live here; ask the Sturgess's — first house west of route 400 on 6th Line — they have been here all their lives."
>
> Mrs. Sturgess said George Little now lives in Hawkestone

(about 5 miles from our own cottage!); he sometimes works at "Driftwood" Restaurant on 400, feeding the animals. Asked there — he works there, but they hadn't his address.

Sept. 1

George Little is listed in phone book. |Phone number and postal address given.| Asked at Hawkestone store where to find him. |Hand-drawn map supplied.|

George Little seems to be no relation of Robert Little and Susannah Cross . . .

Later, Elizabeth and I drove around Innisfil township. We had a picnic near Robert Little's old farm, visited the Innisfil Historical Document Centre

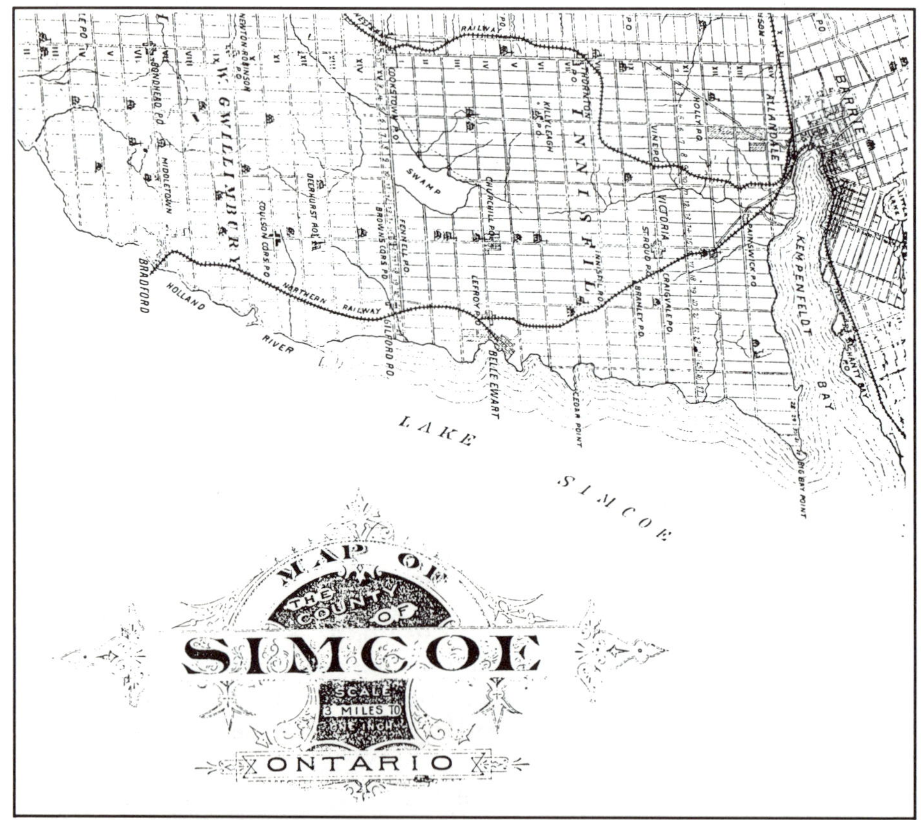

From the Belden Illustrated Historical Atlas of the Dominion of Canada (Simcoe edition) 1881

and talked with members of the Historical Society. Like the people of Warracknabeal, the local historians of Innisfil were enthusiastic, very interested in the project, and eager to help.

The *Historical Review* proved to be a fine example of how helpful can be the simple information compiled by people concerned about keeping some records of the past of their families or communities. The essay on "my" Little family told something about how William C. Little's father and mother had come to the area. It also gave brief resumés of the careers of William and his siblings. I now knew that he was one of eight children. He had one brother (Jim, as I already knew) and six sisters (Mary and Helen, in addition to the ones named in his letters). The girls had married and had families and, fortunately, the *Historical Review* gave some indication of what had happened to their children. For example, one sentence said: "Dr. Lillian Chase in Toronto is a specialist in Diabetics." This information was already thirty years old, but I thought it might be helpful in tracking down the next generation of Littles. Faith Wallis, of McGill's Osler Library, checked and found that Dr. Lillian Chase was still listed in a 1984 Ontario medical directory. I found her phone number, made an appointment and went to see her.

Dr. Lillian Chase was Dr. William C. Little's niece (his sister Elizabeth's daughter). She was therefore a member of "the delightful family named Chase" who had made Jenny Gaff "feel one of the family" in 1910. Indeed, Dr. Lillian, who was ninety-one at the time of my interview, was about sixteen when "Uncle William" visited Nova Scotia. She had actually met him! She remembered him as a dark man without a trace of grey, and she remembered that there was a woman with him. "Perhaps his housekeeper," she suggested tentatively. "No," I said, positively. "That was Nurse Jenny Gaff." Dr. Chase was startled that I should be so certain of such a detail. "This is weird," she said and I had to agree. It must have seemed bizarre to have a complete stranger suddenly appear out of the blue and to be taking an interest in her family, especially an uncle dead so long ago and far away. Be that as it may, for this inquirer, it was a great thrill to meet someone who was not only a close relative of my subject but who had actually met him. Given all the circumstances, the chances of this happening must have been very slim indeed.

○　○　○

Perhaps because Dr. Lillian Chase had lived for two years with her grandparents (W.C.L.'s parents) while she was studying medicine in Toronto, she had been well-attuned to family matters. Her Uncle William was dead by that time, but she must have heard his parents speak of him often. She did not know the "crazy" date of his birth, but she was able to contribute the interesting footnote that Dr. William Clow Little had given himself his second name. All the Little children, she assured me, had been baptized with one name only (as the census record showed). He had added "Clow" himself. That explained why the official registers of Queen's University and the Ontario College of Agriculture had him listed only as "William Little."

Indeed, the information on William Little at Queen's was sparse, as the assistant archivist indicated in response to my original inquiry. The registrar's records told only that he entered Medicine in 1885 and graduated in 1889. They contained none of the usual biographical information such as date of birth, father's name and occupation, or religion. On my subsequent search in the Queen's archives, I was unable to find anything further — apart from seeing "W. Little" listed alphabetically in examination and gradua-tion lists. My visit to Queen's proved more productive of material on his fellow student, Grace Ritchie, or at least on the general question of medical education for women. Dr. A.A. Travill, who had published an extended essay on the Kingston Women's Medical College, was generously willing to share his expert knowledge, as was his colleague, Dr. Sam Shortt, who seemed particularly interested in economic aspects of medical history and hence in the fees Billy Little told Grace Ritchie he charged for his professional services.

The Ontario College of Agriculture held the key to the puzzles posed by the article on Dr. Little in *The Cyclopedia of Victoria* concerning his winning a prize awarded by the Government of Ontario, and being asked by the Government of Canada to bring back selected animals from the royal herds at Windsor Castle. I discovered that the Ontario College of Agriculture had been established (with another name) in 1874, and was under the con-trol of the Ontario Government Department of Education. In the 1960s, it became part of the University of Guelph. I therefore contacted the Archival Section of the University of the Guelph Library, where I was warned that the old records were also "rather sparse." Still, librarians Sarah Funston and Nancy Sadak were imaginative and helpful. In the College Roll for the 1881-82 session we found the following entry:

Name	*P.O. Address*	*County*
Little, W.	Killyleagh	Simcoe

(Killyleagh proved to be the name of the rural post office nearest the Little farm. It no longer exists.)

We also found W. Little's name in the Annual Reports for 1881/82, 1833, and 1883/84. In the 1883 Midsummer Examination Lists we saw he had placed second in Mathematics and been awarded an Honour Certificate. In the 1883 Annual Report, under "Prizes awarded on the Results of the Easter Examinations — First Year," we found the answer to one of the puzzles. W. Little had come first in Agriculture and had won a prize. Technically, he had been awarded a prize by the Government of Ontario!

Then, what about the stock from Windsor Castle? According to the 1884 Annual Report, the Ontario College of Agriculture was involved in the purchase of livestock to improve Canadian herds. The project was under the direction of the Professor of Agriculture and Farm Manager, William Brown. Professor Brown submitted a full, impressively illustrated report on his trip, which involved travelling two thousand miles in Britain, spending more than $25,000, and included selecting animals from the herds at Windsor Castle. There is no mention of W. Little in Professor Brown's report but it is quite reasonable to conclude, as Ms. Sadak did, that "It would be quite possible that able and interested students would have accompanied him." William Little's academic record suggested that he was both "able and interested" and the long trip abroad might explain why he, a very good student, was registered for at least three years for a two-year diploma course. Further, if Professor Brown selected him as an assistant (and perhaps placed him in immediate charge of the livestock on the return journey), then he probably would have received some sort of official communication from the Department of Agriculture approving his participation. Technically, then, William Little would have been asked by the Government of Canada!

Working on this assumption, I wrote to the Public Archives of Canada and, in due course, received a response. Archivist Tom Nesmith informed me that:

> Unfortunately, Professor Brown's trip to Great Britain did not generate correspondence with the Department of Agriculture during the mid-1880s. All is not lost, however! The H.B. Sharman Papers (MG 30 C 224) in the custody of the Manuscript Division of the PAC does contain information pertinent to your inquiry. Sharman was a student at OAC in the 1880s. He and another student, A.W. Ballantyne (according to Sharman's student scrapbook in volume four) accompanied Brown to Great Britain in 1884. There is no mention, though of a William Little. The source in the scrapbook is a newspaper clipping which quotes Brown. I assume that if Little went, he would have been mentioned too.

Tom Nesmith's assumption makes sense. It is likely that if W.C.L. went with Brown, Sharman and Ballantyne, he would have been mentioned. But not necessarily. The evidence remains inconclusive. Perhaps William Little really went with them, or perhaps he only wished he did. Dr. Chase could recall no family anecdote relating to this trip. Further, it does seem very unlikely that the Government of Canada would have asked both Professor Brown and student William Little to undertake two separate trips to Britain for the purchase of livestock. Brown's mission is well substantiated, Little's may only have been a dream and his claim merely a piece of self-aggrandisement. Had I unwittingly called his bluff? If it had seemed ''weird'' for me to know such details of Dr. Little's life as the name of the person with whom he had travelled in 1910, was it downright churlish of me, after so many years to unmask his harmless exaggerations and possibly suggest that my hero might have had feet of clay? Alas, that is all too often a part of the historian's task, a part that must not be neglected or denied.

○   ○   ○

I believe it was because this was essentially a biographical study that "the pursuit of Billy Little" generated an extraordinary amount of voluntary assistance. While it required the generous sharing of time and effort, it appeared to rouse curiosity and to give a good deal of satisfaction to all those who participated in it. For me, the principal investigator, it was an engrossing part-time quest that — to this point — had uncovered much information but had left many questions unanswered.

A second, more extended visit to Australia with more time to read the old Warracknabeal papers, to study the historical background, and to conduct further interviews would be required to fill in the gaps. Then, from all evidence and understanding obtained from inquiries in Canada and Australia, it would be possible to offer some explanatory notes on the letters of William C. Little and Grace Ritchie, and to write reasonable accounts of their lives and times in order to place the letters in context.

Backgrounds

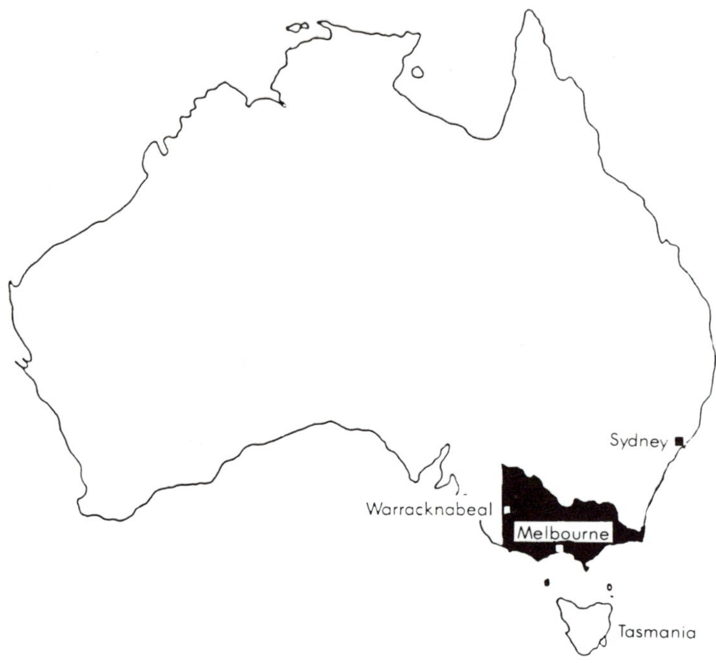

Map of Australia showing Warracknabeal in the State of Victoria

Backgrounds

Ecclefechan in Dumfriesshire has a singularly attractive name, but it is just one of a multitude of Scottish villages that has seen its spirited young people sail off on the high seas seeking fortune and happiness in foreign parts. In 1847, one of these adventurers from Ecclefechan was nineteen-year-old Robert Little, who set off to brave the turbulent Atlantic and become a pioneer in the great wilderness of Canada. He disembarked in Quebec, then journeyed overland to Upper Canada (now Ontario), where he acquired title to land in Innisfil Township. "Township" is perhaps a misleading word, for it does not mean a small settlement so much as a large rural area (in this case, 68,653 acres). The nearest town of any size was Barrie, about three miles away on the shores of Kempenfeldt Bay, Lake Simcoe. The area was described by a fulsome nineteenth-century writer as "a succession of handsome undulations, charming gentle glades, verdure carpeted and forest-flanked, gentle swells revelling in natural and acquired charms of grove and garden and decided eminences . . ."[1] However, Robert Little needed all the Scottish grit and determination he could muster to survive the rigors of snow-bound winters in his hut of roughly-hewn logs and summers of unexpectedly intense heat. He also had to endure isolation and privation from virtually all creature comforts. Yet for all his toughness, Robert Little was a romantic and he made the most of his lot.

This young immigrant may have been isolated, but he did not toil alone in the wilderness, neither was he without the company of other Scots. Indeed, there were many of his countrymen in Upper Canada, including a group who had settled at distant Dalhousie. These were weavers, tradesmen, and artisans — mainly from Glasgow — who had struggled for years to farm around the unyielding rocks of Dalhousie before Governor Simcoe granted them land in the county that bore his name. In the 1830s, these Dalhousie settlers had packed their worldly goods onto unwieldly ox-carts and trekked the many springless, weary miles towards Innisfil Township. Among them was a family called Cross. And one member of that family was a child called Susannah. In her new home, Susannah Cross grew into a healthy, vigorous young woman (indeed, she was to live to a hale ninety-six years). Inevitably, there was more than one young Scots-Canadian man who wished to rescue her from the household chores that filled her days, for her mother took in as boarders men who were building a railroad. Robert Little was among the aspirants for Susan Cross's hand. He knew, however, that he had a serious rival and was not at all sure that his own suit would be favourably received. Neither did he know how to find out what she thought of him nor what his chances were. Then one Sunday as the three of them — Robert Little, Susan Cross and the other young man — were walking home along a bush trail from the Presbyterian church they all attended, Providence sent a sign.

Robert saw that there was a stump blocking the trail ahead so that it would be impossible for all three to pass it together. He said to himself, "If she comes to my side of the stump, it will be a good omen. If she does, I will propose." He must have approached the fateful stump with fluttering heart and passed by it with pulses pounding, for she chose his side. What is more, the omen spoke truly. He proposed and she accepted.

When Robert Little and Susan Cross were married they lived the typical life of the self-sufficient, hardworking settlers in mid-nineteenth-century Upper Canada. They cleared their land, plowed their fields, grew their own food, wove their own cloth, made their own clothes, and turned tallow into candles. Thus, about twenty years after Robert Little had set off from Scotland, he and Susan were the owners of fifty acres, three horses, two carts, six milk cows, eight other cattle, sixteen sheep, and nine swine. In the fullness of time, they also had a great brood of children: six daughters and two sons (Mary, Helen, William, James, Elizabeth, Isabella, Margaret, and Susan). In Scottish tradition, they wanted the best possible education for all their offspring, sacrificing to make their dream a reality. Accordingly, Mary studied oil painting, Helen took music lessons (and played the church organ even to her eightieth year), William and Isabella studied medicine, Elizabeth and Margaret went to normal school to train as teachers, Susan took an arts degree and became the first National General Secretary of the YWCA in Canada, and James became a bookseller, specializing in scientific and medical works. None of the eight children followed their parents onto the land. All the girls married and their families spread across Canada from Nova Scotia to British Columbia, and to the United States. All the young Littles inherited some of the venturesome spirit of their forebears and responded to the allure of distant places. Both boys were to spend the greater part of their lives in Australia. So, in 1890, Robert and Susan sold their farm and went to live in Toronto. Sadly, there was no one to carry on the work they had so enthusiastically begun.

○   ○   ○

At one time William Little had intended to become a farmer. He had gone through secondary school at the Barrie Collegiate,[2] stayed at home for a while working with his parents, and then enrolled at the Ontario Agricultural College (O.A.C.). This was a fairly new institution, established in 1874 by the Ontario Department of Education at Guelph as part of a growing movement in Canada to give systematic, scientific bases to practical farming. The records show that William Little enrolled in the two-year Diploma of Agriculture Course at O.A.C. in 1881. He was then twenty-one years old. The records also show that he was a very good student, that he did particularly well in livestock and mathematics, and that he was registered until 1884. Curiously, they do not list him among the graduates. His apparent failure to graduate in agriculture remains something of a mystery and may be simply a product of the fragmentary nature of the records. It might also be due to the fact that, good student though he was, Billy Little's heart was not in it so that he was not engrossed in his work. He mentions in a letter (August 3, 1890) that, at one point in his life — probably during this period — he "got all wrong, pale and out of sorts." He says that to remedy this condition, he "quit studying and took a sea voyage to Ceylon." This was a rather extraordinary thing for a relatively poor farm boy from Ontario to do a hundred years ago — or even now — but Billy Little was not an ordinary young man.

His prescription proved to be a good one, even if the trip was not entirely successful. He speaks of "dear old Colombo, the place where I went to seek my fortune and didn't find it" (November 25, 1889). If he returned to Canada as poor or even poorer than when he left, he was at least able to say that the voyage "brought back his color, rejuvenated his nerves and gave him a new lease on life." During that Guelph period, it is possible that he travelled to Britain with Professor James Brown and at least two other students to select and bring back to Canada prize livestock from various herds, including the royal herds at Windsor Castle.[3] In any event, he emerged from these years with an excellent knowledge of livestock, a sound basic training in science, and a desire to change his vocation.

William Little had decided to become a doctor. In 1885, when he had reached the mature age of twenty-five, the farmer's son enrolled in the

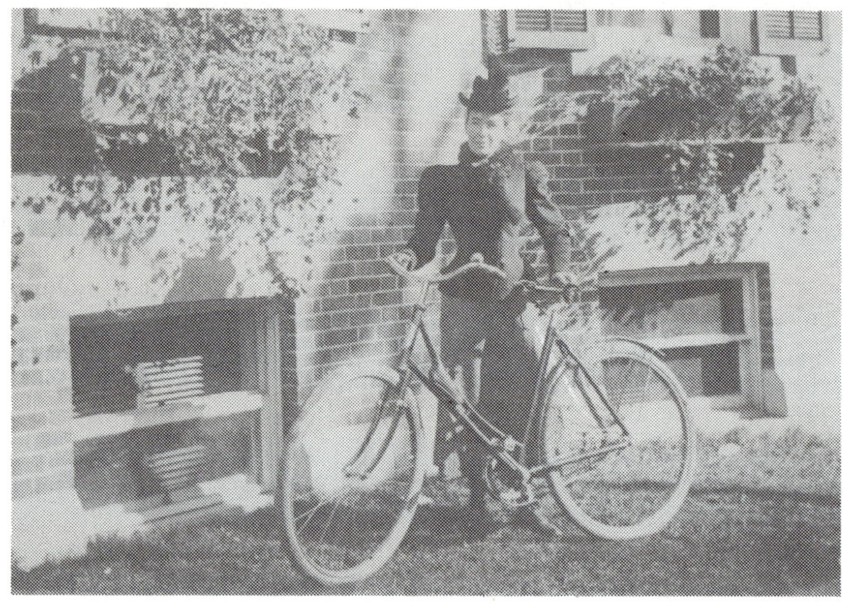

Octavia Grace Ritchie

medical course at the Royal College of Physicians and Surgeons, which was affiliated with Queen's University, Kingston, Ontario. It was here, three years later, that he met Grace Ritchie.

Octavia Grace Ritchie was born in Montreal in 1868, the eighth child of Jessie and Thomas Weston Ritchie. Her father was a lawyer and her ancestors on his side were, like Billy Little's, of Scottish descent; on her mother's side they were of Scottish and United Empire Loyalist stock. Her great, great maternal grandfather, Philip Embury, was a noted Methodist preacher who had been personally inspired by John Wesley. He emigrated from Ireland to New York and in 1776, soon after he had built the first Methodist church in America, he died there. Then, in the wake of the American Revolution, his widow and two children fled north to the safety of Canada. Grace Ritchie, or "Tavie" as she was known at home, was proudly fifth-generation Canadian.

Although she essentially grew up in the Eastern Townships regions of Quebec, she spent two years of her childhood in Germany and later attended the Montreal High School for Girls. When she graduated from that institution in 1884, no women had yet been admitted to degree programmes at Montreal's McGill University; prospects of higher education for her looked dim. However, it was partly due to the excellent results she and some of her classmates earned in the matriculation examinations, together with their determination to undertake further study, that the old order crumbled and she became a member of the first group of women at McGill. She graduated with her B.A. in 1888 and was chosen as valedictorian of that historic first class. Yet her ambitions were still not satisfied, for she wished to study medicine. That is what took her to Queen's.

In the 1880s, Queen's had a growing reputation but it was remarkable for being affiliated with the Kingston Women's Medical College (K.W.M.C.). The K.W.M.C. was one of the first Canadian institutions to offer medical training to women and, not surprisingly, its origins were marked by some fierce controversy. [4] In 1879, thanks to the initiative of a spunky, determined individual, Elizabeth Smith, the Royal College of Physicians and Surgeons had agreed to let women sit its matriculation examinations. Elizabeth Smith was warmly encouraged by her mother, but before she approached the Royal College, she sought support from other women. She placed the following advertisement in the Toronto *Globe:* "Ladies wishing to study medicine in Canada will hear something to their advantage by communicating with Box 31, Winona." Interested responses came from eleven young women and discouraging warnings from a number of other people. One of these, a typical crank letter, read:

> Don't be in a hurry to teach Ladies the 'curious arts' Acts (xix. 19) of sorcery and witchcraft called in scripture Pharmacies upon which Pharmacy is based, get instructed yourself in the greatest revolution in physiology and Materia Medica, known as the Gospel Health Movement.
>
> Yours in the Great Physician Jesus Christ
> Victor B. Hall [5]

In the end, only two other women (Alice McGillivray and Elizabeth Beatty) joined Elizabeth Smith for the special course for women set up at Queen's in the summer of 1880.

These three young women were almost obsessively determined to do well. They studied endlessly and they braced themselves against the gruesome sights of their first operation — the brutality, the blood, the stench. They were resolved not to faint, be sick, uninformed, late or frivolous or anything else that might mark them as unworthy of the serious profession they aspired to enter. They did very well (too well, according to some of the males on campus), but nevertheless the special course was not offered them the following summer. After much cogitation, however, the three women were allowed

1888-'89.

⟶ SIXTH ANNUAL CALENDAR ⟵

— OF THE —

Women's Medical College, Kingston

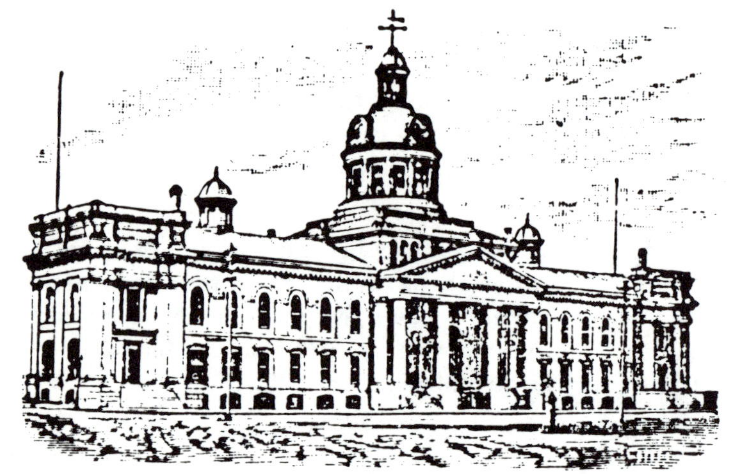

CITY BUILDING—LOCATION OF COLLEGE.

— IN AFFILIATION WITH —

QUEEN'S UNIVERSITY.

KINGSTON, ONT.:
PRINTED AT THE BRITISH WHIG OFFICE,
1888.

into the regular medical course in the autumn of 1881. This was widely acknowledged as an extraordinary experiment in co-education. In general, any form of higher education for women, especially medical education, was a contentious issue throughout the second half of the nineteenth century. Medical co-education was practically unthinkable, for the very idea of nice young ladies studying subjects like anatomy in the presence of young men was horrifying. Still, at the Royal the new venture began peacefully.

To spare blushes all round, the women were assigned to a separate dissecting room, and for some classes, such as obstetrics, they were required to sit in a room adjacent to the main lecture hall. Thus selectively segregated, they passed their first session without major incident. The second year, however, was a disaster. Suddenly, the women became the butt of endless ribaldry, embarrassing anecdotes, bawdy graffiti, and disgusting booby traps. Some male students and some professors made their lives a torture. Physiology classes especially became a dreaded nightmare. The three female pioneers now needed their pluck and grit, and their sense of humour. They called themselves "Shadrack," "Meshach" and "Abednego" because they were going through such fire. Elizabeth Smith wrote in her diary: "No one knows or can know what a furnace we are passing through at College. We suffer torment, we shrink inwardly, we are hurt cruelly." [6]

"Shadrach," "Meshach" and "Abednego," along with the two others who had joined them in the second year, finally could take no more. They went off to the registrar to protest the obscene leers and bawdy remarks of one Dr. Kenneth N. Fenwick, Professor of Obstetrics and Gynaecology, their physiology instructor. The matter then became public, the campus erupted, the male students went on strike, threatening to migrate in a body to Toronto if the Medical Faculty did not get rid of the women. [7] After a great deal of wrangling and the intervention of some prominent citizens of Kingston, a compromise was reached. The women, innocent victims that they were, were not to be expelled but would have to take all their classes quite apart from the men. They would have a separate college, though degrees would still be granted by Queen's. Thus, the Kingston Women's Medical College formally came into being in 1883. Classes were given in the top floor of the City Building downtown, where the facilities were officially described as "commodious" "comfortable" and "convenient," showing "a consideration and appreciation of girl nature very commendable." Within two years, the *Queen's College Journal* noted that ". . . medicals, however much they may dislike the fact of having lady competitors in the same field of study, must now swallow the pill with good grace, since women have proved themselves intellectually equal, in many instances, to men" (XII.1.8). The

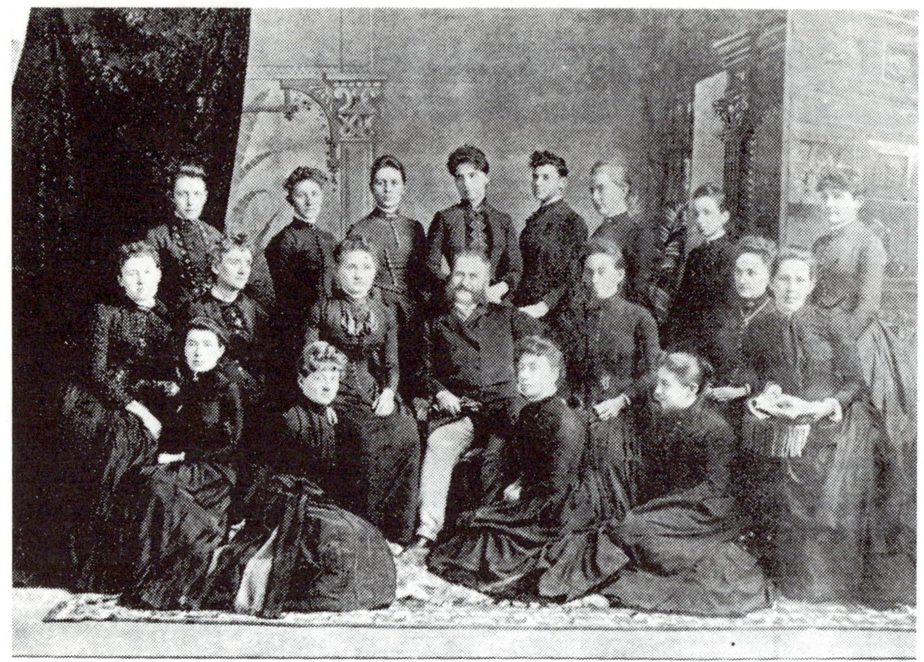

CLASS IN SURGERY 1891, WITH THE DEAN, HON. SENATOR SULLIVAN,
KINGSTON WOMAN'S MEDICAL COLLEGE.

Grace Ritchie far left, front row

K.W.M.C. grew, it appointed some of its first graduates to its staff and, by 1888, the year in which Grace Ritchie arrived from Montreal, it had prepared fifteen women for the degree of M.D., Ch.M. (Even so, the male professors still had difficulty thinking of them professionally and joked that "M.D." stood for "My Darling.")

Grace Ritchie was permitted to register in the second year of K.W.M.C.'s four-year programme because she already held the Bachelor of Arts degree from McGill. She was, of course, entirely in harmony with the views and actions of people like Elizabeth Smith for she, too, had tried to force a formidable institution to admit women to medicine. In the valedictory address she had given at her graduation cermoney she had strongly pleaded for women's rights. "The doors of the Faculty of Arts were opened four years ago; those of Medicine still remain closed. When will they be opened?" she demanded.[8] Her words were greeted with cries of "Never!" and "Shame!" For thirty years McGill would resolutly refuse to admit women to its senior faculty. Therefore, though she would have preferred to stay in Montreal, Miss Ritchie, B.A., wanted to become a doctor as soon as possible and, if that meant going to Kingston to study, to Kingston she would go. So it happened that in the autumn of 1888 she became both a medical student at the K.W.M.C. and a resident at Allen's boarding house, which was located at 40 Stewart Street, Kingston.

○ ○ ○

It was during the 1888-89 academic year that Grace Ritchie and William Little met. He was then a twenty-eight-year-old senior about to graduate, she was an idealistic young woman of twenty who was as determined as Elizabeth Smith to become a doctor. They may have seen each other first strolling on the beautiful Queen's campus, at one of the chaperoned social functions held for students, or at Allen's boarding house. In its day, the boarding house has played an important role in many a romance, and Allen's was no exception. Several other young ladies from the K.W.M.C. — Laura Bennett, Elizabeth Henderson, Clara Demorest, and Hattie Walker — boarded there, so did William Little and some of the other male students from Queen's. What an opportunity this afforded the young people to get together. What a mockery it made of the great efforts the colleges had taken to keep them apart!

Still, the women at Allen's formed a natural alliance against the male college world into which they had "intruded" and they became especially fast friends. In the manner of their day, they gave themselves nicknames, with sobriquets such as "The Whale,""The Hen," and "The Porpoise." Together, that little group became known as "The Menagerie." Billy Little did not seem to harbour any bitter prejudices against lady medical students. Quite the contrary. He had his photograph taken with "The Menagerie" and he kept the picture on his mantle for many years. In a very different context, it brought back nostalgic memories of the good times they all had together during their student days in Kingston. They went on excursions, amused themselves with currently fashionable palmistry and mesmerism, shared lecture notes and made casts of each others' hands. Some of these activities, of course, brought them into close contact and it is not to be wondered if discreet love affairs began over a bowl of plaster of Paris. Perhaps that is where Billy Little's affection for Grace Ritchie was born.

Like his father, Billy Little was a romantic. He felt warmly towards all members of "The Menagerie" but he had his favourites. He confessed to Grace Ritchie (alias "The Porpoise") that he had been in love with Laura Bennett, but she "did not love him in return." Luckily, he was a resilient sort of fellow and recovered his equanimity. Indeed, he fell in love with Grace Ritchie. There is no doubt that his feelings for her were strong and enduring.

His letters attest to this by their existence as well as their content, for no busy person keeps up a lengthy correspondence over five years on the basis of college nostalgia alone. She did not say that she, too, "did not love him in return," but that she was not ready to marry. She wanted to become a doctor in her own right. She saw their careers as running parallel, rather than converging. Many of his letters to her consciously recognize this for, near the signature, there is often a curiously romantic cypher: two parallel lines, the one representing him, the other her. When these parallel lines happened to waver inwards, she surely noticed and commented that they were coming just a bit too close altogether.

Still, Grace kept up her end of the correspondence, writing frequently, often responding to his letters the very day they arrived, and sending him little gifts from time to time. She and Billy clearly could commune across the miles, sharing new ideas and experiences as well as old memories. Probably she, too, proffered little endearments and romantic innuendos. But on another level, Grace Ritchie was intent on keeping her distance. Her resolve to succeed in breaking through the prejudice against women in medicine was unswerving. He respected her for this, for he could see that she "had the material to make a pretty good doctor" (January 23, 1890) and he gave her advice and some of his most favoured prescriptions to help her with her professional development. Her determination to practise medicine was not to be sidetracked, not even when he proposed that she come to Australia to join him. He suggested that they might put out their shingle with a legend that read, not "Drs. Little and Ritchie," but "Drs. Ritchie and Little." She seems to have countered with something like, "I want my $50,000 practice first." It is anyone's guess what she said in answer to his gambit, "I have taken such a liking to riding, I gave a special prize or part of one for the best lady rider. Won't you come and try for it?" The parallel lines continued.

Special Prizes.

2. High jumper, to take such leaps as the judges may direct. First prize, £16; second, £4; third, £2; fourth £1.

3. Weight-carrying hackney, up to 12 stone. First prize, £5; second, £2; third £1. Silver watch value £5 5s (the gift of Eliza Tinsley, Melbourne), to the best gentleman rider.

4. Light hackney. First prize, £2; second, double reined bridle (the gift of G. P. Fergie, Warracknabeal), value 25s; gentleman's riding whip (the gift of W. F. Schickerling, Warracknabeal), value 21s, to be awarded to the best rider.

5. Lady's hunter to take such leaps as judges may direct. First prize, £5; second, £2. Best equestrienne in this section. First prize £5 (£3 the gift of Dr. Little, Warracknabeal, and £2 the gift of J. J. Still, Warracknabeal); second, £3 (the gift of Messrs. Hicks, Grace and Bell, Warracknabeal.)

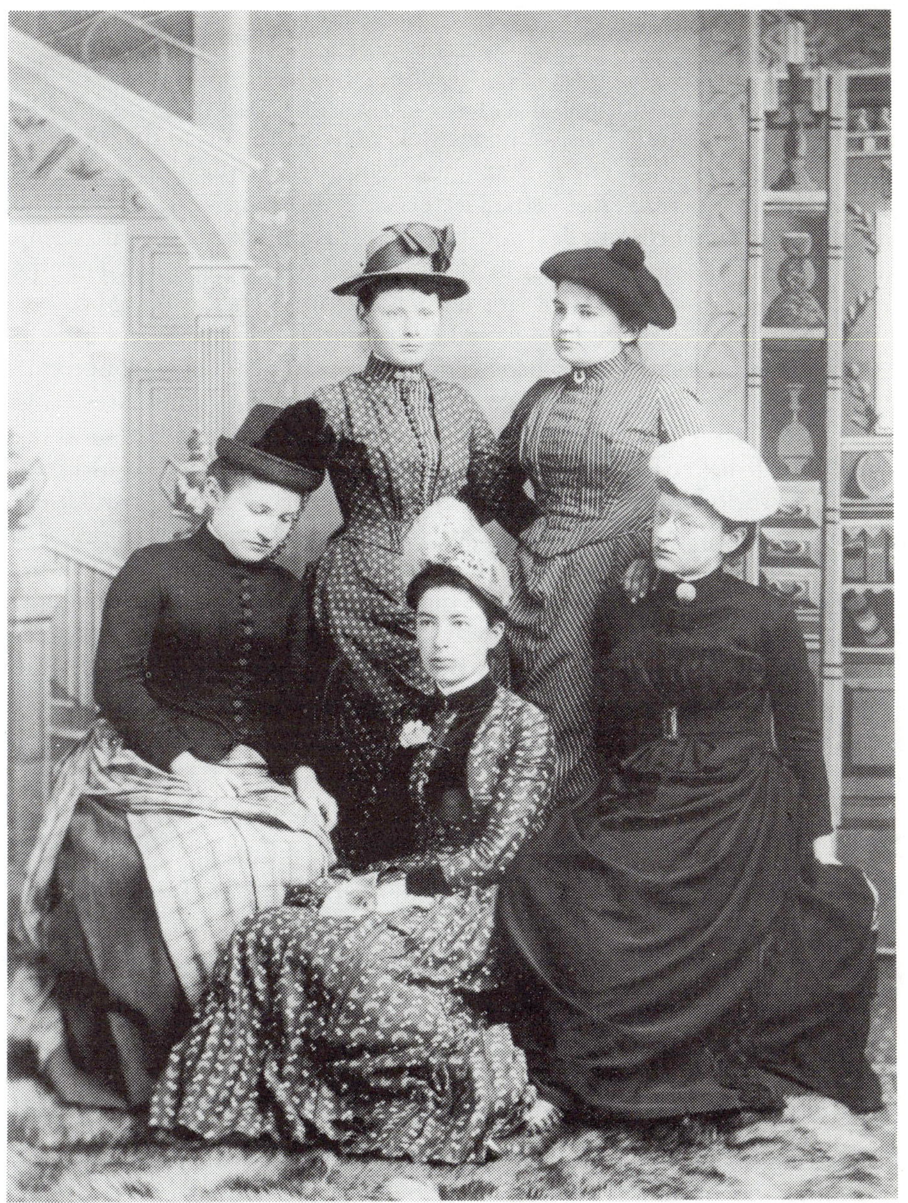

Grace (C), Maude Abbott (top R) and friends

In the spring of 1889, William C. Little graduated from Queen's College with his M.D., Ch.M. Degree. At some point during his medical studies he had acquired a middle name, Clow. This was apparently an old family name that, incidentally, his younger sister, Isabella, the other doctor among his siblings, also adopted. Perhaps he thought a middle initial gave him a touch of distinction, just as the letters after his name did. He was not, however, overwhelmed by his newly won status and was content to enjoy life, spending the early summer in Montreal and seeing a good deal of Grace Ritchie. He met members of her family, including her sister, Mrs. Jessie Savage, and her close, life-long friend, Maude Abbott. Maude Abbott, then a rather large young woman who cheerfully accepted her grossly inappropriate nickname, "The Fairy," was also among the early McGill graduates in Arts (B.A. '91). Like Grace, she was keen on becoming a doctor. Her ambitions were to be fulfilled, for she not only got her medical degree but ultimately earned a world-wide reputation for her work on congenital heart disease. That, however, was well into the future. During that interlude of '89, these young people relaxed in Montreal and environs, making trips to the Eastern Townships. Grace Ritchie had spent many a happy time there, enjoying the countryside, the hills and the waterways such as Lake Massawippi — a curious Amerindian name and a word that Billy Little was to recall when he sought a name for his private hospital in distant Australia.

○   ○   ○

All too soon, Dr. Little had to make an important decision about his future. In order to practise medicine in the province of Ontario, he would have to pass the exams of the Ontario Council of Physicians and Surgeons or obtain a licence from a recognized overseas body. Like many Canadians of his time, he chose to go to Britain and, because of the fame of Edinburgh in the medical world, he set off for Scotland. It seems he followed Grace Ritchie's advice, studied hard, and took the examinations of the Royal College of Surgeons, Edinburgh, as soon as he could. The present correspondence with Grace begins as he reports to her that he has been successful in getting the Licentiate. He tells her about it with a mixture of pride, humility and humour, claiming that the secret of passing oral exams is to smile and appear confident. This formula certainly worked for him. His distinguished examiners may have thought him a brash young colonial, but they apparently appreciated his ingenuity in improvising a way to deal with a scalp wound, and his honesty in confessing that he had never seen a Coudé catheter, one of the instruments he was asked to describe.

By the autumn of 1889, after some relaxation, visits to relatives, a brief, eye-opening encounter with the Edinburgh slums, and a trip to London, Dr. Little was ready to start on his life's work. He had decided to practise medicine in Australia. Why Australia?

It is pretty clear from the first letter that W.C.L. did not really know a great deal about the country. For example, he referred to the native people as Maoris rather than Aborigines, and it was a while before he understood that a pickaninny was a young aborigine. But it is also clear that he was thinking about Australia while he was in Edinburgh. There were several possible inducements for him to have done so and for him to consider going so far away from home.

First of all, the travelling and the distance would not necessarily have posed great obstacles to an ambitious young man who wanted to see the world. There was a strong tradition of travel, adventure and enterprise in his immediate family, as well as in his general background or what has been called "the Scottish diaspora."[9] This tradition could, at least, make the extremely long and uncomfortable journey from Britain to Australia thinkable. Beyond that, he personally enjoyed travel and the discovery of new places. He said once that if he had the means "there is not a country or people in the world but what I would see." He wondered in writing to Grace, "What is the good of going to heaven ignorant of the earth?" (August 3, 1890). Furthermore, a trail to Australia had already been blazed. W.C.L. knew a surprising number of people there, both friends and relatives. His younger brother, James, had already been there for two years. Billy noted that both he and James had "roving dispositions." James travelled a good deal in Australia but was eventually to marry, settle down, have a family of four children and open a medical and scientific bookshop at 263 Collins St.,

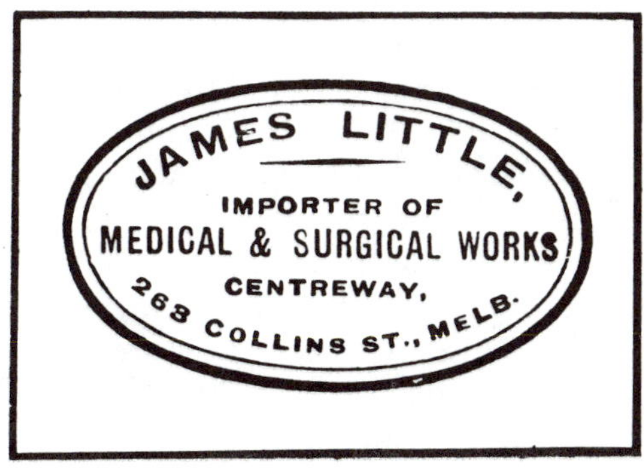

Melbourne. Then there was his cousin, Dr. William Joseph Cross. He had taken a medical degree at the University of Toronto in 1879 and his Licentiate at Edinburgh the following year, had sailed off for Australia and, in 1881, had established a successful medical practice at Horsham, Victoria. Yet another cousin, Dr. James Allan Cross, who had his M.D., Ch.M. from Victoria College, University of Toronto, was in London in 1889 reading for his Licentiate of the Royal College of Surgeons there. It is more than likely that when Dr. William C. Little came down from Edinburgh to visit London that year, he and his cousin, Dr. James Cross, would have discussed their plans and the apparent satisfaction Dr. William Cross was finding in Australia. It could hardly be a coincidence that James Cross also migrated to Australia, where he went into practice in Murtoa, Victoria, towards the end of 1890.

Probably James Little and William Cross wrote to their kinfolk with attractive descriptions of their new country but, if not, there were plenty of other sources of information. W.C.L., who was a keen reader, might well have encountered popular reference works such as *The Australasian Medical Directory and Handbook* compiled by Ludwig Bruck. This was first published in 1883 and ran through several editions. It contained lists of medical practitioners, obituaries, medical societies, scales of fees, and regulations affecting the profession, as well as a general gazetteer and road guide. In a word, it had everything anyone contemplating working as a doctor in mainland Australia, Tasmania or New Zealand might want to know. W.C.L. easily might have consulted the *Directory* and been enticed to the colony of Victoria by Bruck's glowing account of it:

> The climate of Victoria is very similar to that of the more favoured portions of Southern Europe, such as Madrid in Spain, Marseilles, Bordeaux and Nice in France and Bologna and Verona in Italy; however the difference between the coldest and warmest months is much less in Melbourne than in any of these places . . . .The suddenness of the atmospheric changes is felt by some to be trying, but as a rule the climate in autumn, winter and spring is exceedingly agreeable; the atmosphere is transparent, dry and exhilarating. The sky is brightly blue, and soft breezes breathe a delicious freshness and temper the rays of the sun. Even the summer is not oppressively warm, and the dry heat, being cooled by the southerly and south-westerly winds, is rather stimulating . . . . On the whole, Victoria has probably one of the finest climates in the world . . . (pp.134-4).

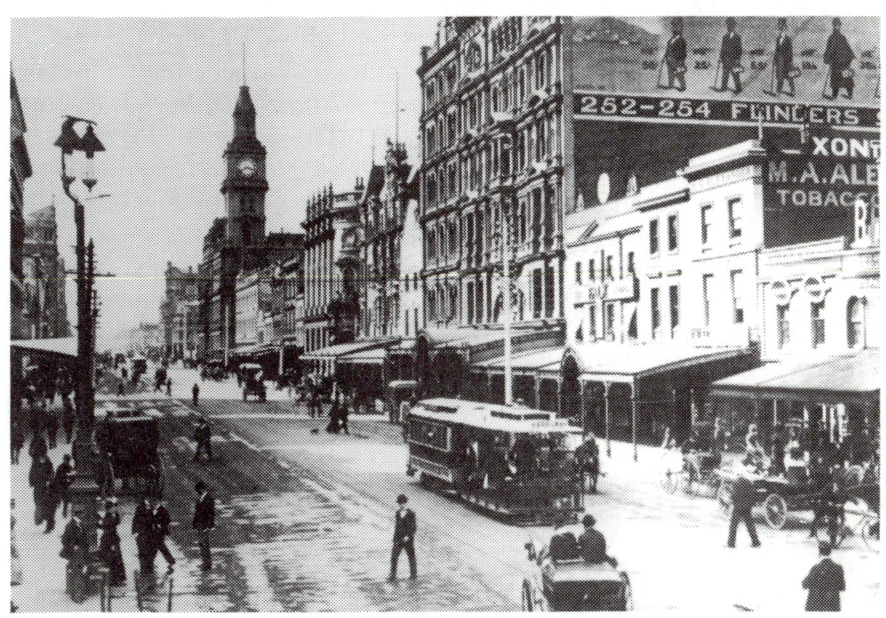

Melbourne circa 1890

No modern glossy tourist brochure could have done much better in lauding the state and, after reading Bruck, any young man with the world at his feet might want to take off in the direction of Victoria.

Furthermore, Victoria's reputation was still infused with the aura of gold. Great discoveries of the precious metal in the middle of the century had made Victoria the most populous of the Australian colonies with more than a million people — including well over a thousand Canadians. Gold had transformed Victoria's major town into "Marvellous Melbourne" with its handsome mansions, fine wide streets, gracious parks and well-stocked shops. In 1889, William Little could not know that the '90s would turn out to be a time of depression. He doubtless saw Australia as a place for rich experience and worthwhile financial rewards. He did not see it as a permanent home, but intended to make his fortune and return to Canada. He thought he would be back in time to go to the great Chicago Exhibition of 1893.

○ ○ ○

Dr. William Clow Little sailed from Southampton aboard the *Kaiser Wilhelm II* on October 6, 1889. His first glimpses of Australia seemed to have coincided pretty well with Bruck's version of the country. In Adelaide he found the people friendly and he "felt at home immediately." On closer acquaintance, his views more nearly matched those of other nineteenth-century visitors to Australia's shores. In 1873, Dr. Walter Richardson (the model for Henry Handel Richardson's Richard Mahony) had described Australia as "that far country where . . .no one speaks without swearing and almost everyone gets drunk." [10] An English novelist, Christie Murray, in 1891 "declared the Australian nation to be one of the most prosperous, educated, rowdy and drunken among the peoples of the world. The country is filled with a feverish, reckless energy with everybody hurrying to be rich. Commercial morality is lax." [11] Billy Little might not have gone that far, but his first tour around Victoria gave him much to think about. He told Grace that while he still had an open mind, he was "not a bit in love with Australia. There is a decided want of moral tone everywhere. Drinking and its accompanying evils are found in all parts. There is an awful lot of looseness, free and easy style amongst both sexes . . . . The climate is such that people have to drink something and soft drinks are not always chosen, as may be noticed on the street every night. The water is not good and the report that typhoid germs are in it give sufficient excuse for not drinking it . . . ." (January 23, 1890). However, the longer he stayed in Australia, the more he got to know it, the more comfortable he felt about it. He even got to the point where he could say, "I am getting to like Australia much better than Canada" (September 28, 1890) and "This is a very nice country and I want you to see it" (November 30, 1890).

All in all, Australia proved to be a pretty good choice of a place for Dr. Little to begin his medical career and he felt that "he landed on his feet" by going there. He was to find that Bruck was right when he had said in the *Australasian Medical Directory* that "The principal diseases prevalent in Victoria are enteric fever, diarrhoeal diseases, diphtheria, pneumonia, phthisis [12] and heart disease" (p.135). He was also to find that his own hopes for working hard and doing well were to be fulfilled. On more than one occasion, with a warm, non-venal kind of glee, he told Grace about the fees he was able to charge and he felt that he was more successful and had more prestige in Australia than he would have had in Canada. But he still intended to go home when the time was right.

To begin his career, Dr. Little acted as a *locum tenens* for his cousin, Dr. William J. Cross, at Horsham in the north-west region of Victoria. This introduction to the district proved quite satisfactory so, before long, he set up his own practice only forty-five miles away. He chose a little town with a big name, Warracknabeal — which means "Place of the Big Red Gums." Then, as now, Warracknabeal was on the Wimmera Plains at about three hundred and sixty feet above sea level. It was an agricultural and pastoral district, an area that has been described as "bare and quiet, intensely flat except for the winding belts of trees in the depressions which in winter are sheeted with fresh rain water and in summer with a glittering mirage." [13] Parts of it were still home to some tribal aborigines when Dr. Little arrived at the beginning of 1890, and the town itself was scarcely twenty years old. It had grown up from being a wayside village, little more than a meeting place for pioneer squatters and settlers, to become a thriving town of "not far short of two thousand" people. [14] The numbers swelled appreciably during harvest and shearing times when brawny, rowdy seasonal workers poured into town. Like the pioneers in Canada, the earliest settlers had had to contend with isolation, loneliness, physical privations and, not cold, but heat. As they had prospered through the growing of wheat and the raising of sheep, as they used innovative farm methods and invented new farming machinery, their town became an important centre with an imposing and busy rail station.

The town was well laid out but, when Billy Little first saw them, the streets of Warracknabeal were still unpaved and rutted by the heavily loaded bullock drays that hauled the bagged wheat to the station. Along Scott Street, the main thoroughfare, there were already substantial commercial buildings of wood and brick, their verandahs elaborately decorated with iron filigree, the elegant "Victorian lace" still found on many buildings throughout the state. The relatively plentiful water supply came from the sleepy Yarriambiac Creek that passed through the edge of town. The creek was not only a source of drinking water, but also the place where people and cattle bathed and where garbage was casually disposed. This was obviously a public health hazard, as were other problems, such as the occasional carcass of a dead animal that was allowed to remain in the main street for a week, becoming, as a local paper put it, "an object of disgust and loathing." [15] Similarly the sewage system was declared to be "a monstrosity."

Clearly, there was work a-plenty for a civic-minded young doctor to do. The nearest public hospital was at Horsham but, by 1891, Warracknabeal was to have its own district hospital. There were two other physicians practising in the town. One of these Dr. Little could count as a colleague, the other was a victim of a fairly wide-spread affliction among Australian doctors, drug taking. Billy Little easily recognized that such a man would pose no threat, be no competition for him.

If the doctor's professional prospects seemed fine in Warracknabeal, his social calendar also appeared likely to be pleasantly crowded. Apart from the natural hospitality that would be showered on him by the people of an Australian country town, there would be opportunities for varied recreational activities through organizations such as the Agricultural Society, the Tennis Club, the Athletic Club, the Racing Club, the Loyal Orange Lodge, and the Caledonian Society. As an attractive, single professional man of thirty, William C. Little could expect to be much in demand in Warracknabeal.

○   ○   ○

The letters that William Little wrote from Warracknabeal are a tiny mirror of life a century ago, giving both the reality of Australia and recollections of Canada. Most of all, they are the personal communications of a young man entering the fullness of his profession to the woman with whom he wanted to share his future. They are rich in personality, discreet in passion.

What a good thing that Grace Ritchie was such a hoarder, that she rarely seemed to throw anything away, that she kept Billy Little's letters. What a pity hers to him are nowhere to be found. If they were not destroyed on some nameless moving or clean-up day, they doubtless disappeared into the flames on the "crematory day once every three months in which all answered correspondence was committed to the flames . . ." (June 8, 1893). So we must be content with reconstructing her side of the correspondence from his responses. Luckily, he wrote so fully that we are left with unique glimpses of the life of a country doctor in the Victoria of the late nineteenth century. More than that, we are privileged to share with Grace Ritchie the encouragement, humour, professional concern, common sense and love of an extraordinary ordinary man, Billy Little.

The Letters
1889-1894

The text of the letters has been reproduced with Billy Little's own sometimes idiosyncratic spelling and syntax. Readers, like Grace, are asked to "overlook whatever they may see amiss" (June 8, 1893).

Grace usually noted the date on which his letters were received (rec.) and when she replied (ans.).

The Letters
1889-1894

(rec. 31 August 1889)

No. 6 Marchmont Crescent,
Edinburgh, July 29/89

My dear Grace,

Your lovely long letter of the 1st instance came to hand some 13 days ago. I was very glad to hear from you. I must compliment you for writing such a lengthy letter. Don't be afraid to write me a long letter for I quite enjoy the reading of them. When you are far from home letters from friends are like "water to a thirsty soul."

I have good news to tell you. I took your advice. I went up for the Exam for "Licentiate of the Royal College of Surgeons of Edinburgh" on the 25 to 27 inst. and I am happy to say that I passed all right. I am now William C. Little, M.D., Ch.M., M.C.P.S.O., L.R.C.S.E. [1] Heavings! what a string to tack onto a "Little" name. The M.D. will answer me for all practical purposes. The written exam was on 25 & the oral yesterday. We had a hard paper on Surgical Anatomy. For e.g., give the minute dissection of the sole of the foot down to the bones. Give the origin, course, relations & points where the Lingual Artery can be ligated etc. I found no difficulty with the questions, only I found when I came home that I had left two muscles out — the transverse pectus and lumbricales. I had a Clinical Exam of one hour in the hospital. The great Jas. Bell and Dr. Craig fired questions at me. I had to do up a Colles fracture [2] and had to cut out the splints. I had to diagnose two cases & got both right but one was a pure guess for I could not make much sense out of the man as he would keep changing his story every minute. When I related the history of the case to Bell and gave him my diagnosis, he slapped his knee and said, "You're right." Imagine my feelings! Was that *Luck?* The House surgeon told me afterwards that the Fellowship men who had been up the day before could not make out the case. The oral exam yesterday was very nice. Dr. Miller and Dr. Somebody-else had a good laugh at me. I was asked in the treatment of a certain case what kind of a Catheter I would use? I told them a "Coudé Catheter." They said I was right & they wanted to know what it was made of. I told them I didn't know, that I never saw one. I thought the Dr. Somebody would have gone into convulsions. With that one answer I got both those men on my side and I just had a fine time with them. Dr. Miller then took me on scalp wounds and asked me how I would treat them. I told him that would just depend on how I was situated. If I had no needles or sutures I would just cleanse the wound & bring the edges together by tying the hair on each side. Miller said he had tried that but the knots in the hair would not hold. I told him I would put wax or gum on the hair first. The two Drs. just sat and stared at me. "Well," said Miller, "I never tried that." I could actually feel my big toes laughing at them but kept a very sober face. The wax or gum just struck me at that moment.

As luck would have it, they then questioned me on the very work I had carefully read the night before. After the thing was all over & I signed my name on the register, Dr. Jas. Bell shook hands with me and wished me success in life. Dr. Miller came & shook hands and said, "You made a splendid Exam in Surgery." I felt like saying, "Come off the roof, if you had just taken me to the wrong place you could have bothered the life half out of me." Still it is very nice to have Examiners speak kindly to you. Thank the Lord I had not an old brute by the name of Watson to examine me. I am sure we would have had a quarrel. He is the most overbearing sarcastic pig in Edinburgh. One of the Canadian students of last year told him to "Go to h—" which was not a gentlemanly thing to say or a nice place to send him. But really I think it is good enough for him. Dr. McEwan, whom you met in Kingston, failed on the exam [that] Duff Rankin and Emery went up for. He told the Examiners he didn't care as he had a better degree than they could give him, that he only wanted it as a trophy to take home. Did you ever hear a more childish speech? I think I have said quite enough about Exams.

Dr. Fenwick was here some two weeks ago. I spent a very pleasant forenoon with him. He advised me not to bother with Exams as it was only a waste of time. Some publisher here has offered to take 150 copies of his book.[3] That speaks well for Fenwick & the Royal. You will find his book will give all the necessary information to pass any exam in Canada or here, still you want a longer work for reference.

I have changed my apartments — have no high stairs to climb. No danger of my heart now as I am on the lower flat. I have a lovely place. I wish you could look in & see me as I am writing. I have a lovely coal fire in the grate & two large easy chairs. I just feel the picture of content. There are some 18 pictures hanging on the wall. One of them I look at quite often. It is Nelson bidding his mother a first farewell. How lovingly she is looking at him as if she were offering up a prayer for his protection from temptation. Another winter scene interests me.

My landlady decided to take holidays, hence my change. I pay 8/- per week for the rooms & have to order whatever I want to eat. Well I never was so badly stuck in my life as I was the first few days. The servant would come in and ask what she would order for dinner. I really did not know how much meat, butter etc. I could eat. I told her to get just what she thought would be enough. I have fattened up a great deal weighing lbs. 170 but I am not a hog, I could not eat half or ¼ [of] what she bought for me. My bill for this week came to £ 1.6/4d. I have learned the price of things at any rate — butter 36cts per lb., meat 18, etc. You guessed my feelings pretty well for I have not seen, heard or tasted a piece of Pie since I left Montreal. I indulge in strawberries, gooseberries and cherries, & a cold bath every morning which makes up for the *pie.*

I miss the Piano as I often whiled away lonesome time by making a noise. I never thought I could learn to play until I found by practising I could get to play a few pieces so that you would recognize them at any rate. There is a violin in the house. I got it on Sunday & was playing some hymns when a milk girl happened to pass. She put down her cans and ran back a short distance & called to another girl that — "Here's a *mon* playing the fiddle on Sunday." Horror was depicted in her face.

I was at the closing exercises of a young ladies' college last week. I had quite a nice time. Some three weeks ago I was at a wedding in St. Giles. A friend sent me a ticket of admittance. The bride looked perfectly lovely & the groom terribly nervous but pleased as well.

Since writing you last I found my cousin, R.E. Little, whom you heard me speak of while in Lachute.[4] Well, I must say I am quite proud of him. He is tall, good-looking and clever. I never saw him before. He has just passed his 2nd professional Exam in the university medical college. He hopes to graduate next spring. I had a most interesting time with him one day as he was going his rounds looking after some poor patients in the Cowgate.

Dear me, what poverty, filth, drunkeness and all that is degrading I witnessed. We went up 6 & 7 flights of stairs to see sick children. Just fancy a family of 5–6–8 living in a room no larger than the little room I had in Kingston. Scarcely a ray of sunlight ever enters these places. The Mothers of the miserable half-starved children were invariably drunk or partially so. Why providence allows such people to have the bringing up of children is more than I know. How true what your friend Miss Birmingham said, "We are all creatures of circumstances." After spending some three hours in this way I became desperate. I said to my cousin, "If you know of anything any worse than I have seen for heavings sake let me see it." "Oh yes," he said, "I can show you places 10 times worse than anything you have seen yet." I would not attempt to put it on paper what I saw and heard. I look on it as my experience while taking a trip through Hell. You said in your last [letter] that men are worse than women because they have greater power to be so. Granting such to be the case, they then have greater power to prevent themselves from becoming so degraded in vice as women. I never knew this before but am satisfied of it now.

My cousin has gone home for a while and is then going to spend his holidays on the Isle of Man. He wants me to go with him but I have not time. He told me his uncle attended the Edinburgh University the same time the Prince of Wales did and that the Prince would often sell his mother's letters for £1 when he was short of cash. Quite an idea.

I think I shall soon spend a week with my friends in the country. I am feeling tired of work. I never worked so faithfully in my life as I have done here. My brain feels tired. I slept nearly all Sunday & did not rise this morning until 11 o'clock.

I have done very little reading outside of medicine. I have met so many interesting cases, so much new work that I have been kept reading all my spare time. I have invested in quite a No. of new books. Oh, by the way, I owe you an apology. You remember in my 1st letter promising to send you a book. Well, after looking it over carefully I concluded you would not like it. It is a little hand book on practical surgery, but dealing altogether with men so I thought you might not like me to send you such a book. If I thought you would like it I would be pleased to give it to you. The part that struck me on looking through it at first was! — to take a cast of the hand for instance. The way to take [it] is the way I suggested, by taking one half at a time. I have thought several times that I was a little bit slow or we could have taken a cast nicely in Lachute.[4] But then you know I was not acquainted with your sister & did not know what she would think of me wanting such a thing. Things like that are very nice if just the two of us only know about it. Any more to know of it would spoil the effect. Don't you think so?

I mailed you some views of Edinburgh last week. I hope you rec. them all right. I hope you rec. the charts all right. They will be of little use to you this year. If you mount them on paste board, do it this way. Cut the card the right size & then rub one side all over with a *"boiled potato,"* boil the potato with the skin on and then peel ½ of it. You have the other ½ for a handle. The Brain chart is worth framing. You can hang one of the charts at a time over your wash stand & when you are dabblng in the water like a little Duck, you can look up & see how your heart is or if you have any of the mentioned symptoms. I had quite a time getting Dr. Sommerville to give them to me. I told him they were for a friend in Canada. He wanted to know if *He* was coming over here. I said I thought he was and that *He* would be likely to attend his class. He then handed them over to me. I would have liked to secure a set for Mrs. Walker, but couldn't. I have not heard from Mrs. Walker. I wrote her from Montreal & gave her my address, but I suppose the poor woman has too many other things to occupy her mind. Still I think she might have sent me a card at any rate.

I have a very useful little book on Surgical Anatomy, one that I used for the Council & here also. I shall mail it to you & will you be good enough to mail it to Mrs. Walker. It is a legacy to be handed down to my friends. Mrs. Walker and Miss Demerest[5] can use it for the Council next spring after which they have to give it to *you* for the Council the following spring & you in turn give it to Miss Henderson. Oh, have you heard from Miss Henderson? Do you think it possible that she is married or that the Napanee trip so disgusted her of this world that she has shut herself up in some harem or convent?

So your brother-in-law was really feeling jealous. Dear me, I am forever getting into trouble of some kind. You should be more careful and not expose me to such dangers. The way I feel about such things is if I admire a lady and another gentleman admires her also, I admire his admiration and feel satisfied that in one thing he is sensible if nothing more. This of course refers to people living in single blessedness.

When I was at the boarding house I made a horrible discovery, my hair nearly stood on end, the cold perspiration stood out in big red drops, my face turned a ghastly blue green as I imagined the police fastening the cold iron handcuffs on my wrists. The cause of all this was on opening the door of a little closet, I discovered the skeleton of a little infant. What was I to do?

I spent the greater part of an afternoon in the Royal Surgeons' Museum. I have often read of tricks of nature but here I had the interesting pleasure of seeing them. I am glad I am not a freak of nature. I saw several mummified heads of Australian Maories. Fancy me marrying one of those horrid looking old things. I would come back to Canada and turn her to good account by making her stand around the streets to make people sick & furthermore I would send her to other Drs. to be treated in order to make them sick so that I would get all the practice.

If you have got over the shock about the infant skeleton I shall finish it. The skeleton is in a glass globe. It was left by a student some years ago. It is all articulated. I have serious intentions of appropriating it as it is just as good as a large one. I fancy it is some two years old.

Did you get as excited as you did over Miss Bennett's yarn?[6]

What a satisfaction it is to feel that I have already written a longer letter than you. This is the longest I ever wrote in my life.

Miss Squire was the lady I saw at the boat. I don't blame your brother for liking her.

So you had the pleasure of an interview with a Woman's Rights [advocate]. Really I don't know what a WR means, but I have an idea it is a woman grown mannish from which good Lord deliver me.

Don't think I had the slightest idea of you becoming such a creature. Oh no! I have quite a number of real interesting pictures of you and in none of them do you figure as a horrid woman's rights [person].

Women have greater powers than men in many ways if they only use them properly. A woman by tact and kindness can lead a man where she will, but let her try to drive him and she will fail for she has taken up weapons that were never intended for her use and she has not the necessary powers to use them.

I had a lovely letter from Dr. Robertson alias "Jack" this morning. He is getting along very well. He would just love to be over here with me and I should like very much to have him here.

You can scarcely imagine my feelings now as my college days are over. I have a feeling of sadness running through me. I am now feeling anxious to get to work. Just where my field of labor will be I cannot say. I am waiting to hear from my brother as to the prospects in Australia. I have met some fine gentlemen from Australia. They say there are lots of good openings but — awful hard work, having to drive 50 and 100 miles. I am fond of driving but not quite so much as that. As soon as I find that my expenses are greater than the income I shall take my departure for Australia. If I go to Australia, can we ever meet again I wonder. Do you intend coming over here to study after you get through at Kingston? There is one more Exam I would like to take here, but I have to be in practice two years before I would be allowed to go up for it. It is the F.R.C.S.E., said to be the best degree in Scotland. The Edinburgh men say L.R.C.S.E., which I have just passed, is as good as the M.R.C.S. of London. Now if I get along well I may come here again in two years and try and get the F.R.C.S.E., merely for the honour of having it. At present I purpose giving my attention to the Eye & Skin. I like Eye surgery but as my Eyes are delicate I could not think of making it a speciality.

I heard quite a nice lecturer on Eczema. Among the causes, he mentioned the use of Arnica as being an exciting cause so be careful about using that pair combination of oil Ricinus and Arnica.

If you are consulted about eczema of the hands or scalp when the skin is dry and scaly order *Starch* poultices. Take a pint of Starch and add a teaspoonful of Boracic acid, apply the poultices until the skin is nice and soft and then wash the part with Anna's fatty Soap or Sapo Viridin and apply some ointment as zinc ox., or Lassers paste. The reason I mention the above is that I was often consulted about eczema or saltrheum as it is generally known and I did not know what to do. If you remember the starch poultice & fatty soap you will be rewarded by getting good results & people will of course think you know all about it: — Anatomical pointer! — Long subscapular nerve supplies latissimus dorsi muscle. Medulla Subscapular nerve Teres Major, Short-subscapular nerve subscapularis. Do you see the point? L. for Latissimus, M. for Major, S. for Subscapularis. Don't forget this.

July 30th

The mail does not go out until tonight and as I got tired writing yesterday I saved this sheet for today. I do not know what has got into me, I want to sleep all the time now. I had a lovely game of Lawn Tennis yesterday evening and went to the opera afterwards, the first opera I have seen since I came here. I am going to have a regular good time for a few days.

I had a letter from Wm. Fair this morning. He tells me Burns of the Kingston P.O. is in the penitentiary. You remember the man you said held the pen so funny. The authorities have issued a writ to arrest Shannon who shipped out a year ago. I cannot understand why old men who have plenty of money should want to steal.

Your postal card came to hand. I am sorry you did not meet Mr. S. I thought he had gone home or had been up to Barrie for I rec. a letter from my cousin, Dr. Cross of London, England, and the first lines were "Hello, Will! I hear you are all broken up on a lady not 1000 miles from Montreal."

Mr. Fair tells me that his little daughter is considered by experts to be a most excellent young one. I would not be at all surprised. Oh, you told me a deadly secret. Well, I shall tell you one far more deadly and you must not ever whisper it in your dreams. Keep awfully still and I shall tell you ——— Jack Duff is all broken up, completely over head and heels in Love with a very fine Edinburgh lady. He was badly smitten and had no means whereby he could get acquainted, so he came and asked me what he would do. I told him if I wanted to get acquainted with a lady and could not get an introduction I would simply write her a note, enclose my card and inform her that I would consider it a great pleasure to make her acquaintance. She then could act as she thought best. Well, Jack wrote her a letter — not a note, a long letter and really he almost told her that he was so much in love with her that he could think of nothing else. The young lady sent him a very nice reply and with her mother's consent invited him to afternoon tea. Now he is happy. Before Jack told me he insisted that I would give my opinion of a young lady that was walking ahead of us on Princess St. I must say I was very favourably impressed but of course as I had not an opportunity to use the *science of Palmistry* I could not tell him all her *good qualities*. This young lady is about 19, just finished at College, is a good musician, good looking, very witty and is in possession of a very honest face, besides she is wealthy. Now be sure and don't mention this in Kingston or it will come right back to me. This affair was not all one-sided as she had taken a fancy to Jack. It is mutual, which makes it just lovely.

Please don't think me a crank writing you such a long letter and if you find any very stupid things in it remember I have been sleeping about 16 hrs. a day since the Exam, which has made my brain feel as if it were dislocated. I shall send "The Devil's Due" if I can place my hands on it: I could not find it in one of the large book stores; however I shall try again.

Now, don't study too hard. Remember a healthy body and an average brain full will bring greater happiness than an overcrowded brain attached to a broken down constitution. It will always be a pleasure for me to assist you in any way that I can. If writing shop interests you, you will find this letter a bit so-so.

Kindly remember me to Mrs. Savage.[7] Ask her if she can turn a buggie around yet. So good bye and remember:

Seas may divide us now yet sunder not
They are not absent — who are not forgot.

Sincerely your friend
William C. Little

P.S.   I have just returned from the infirmary. I had the pleasure of meeting Dr. McGillivray — Dr. Alice.[8] She is over for the good of her health. That fall she got out of the buggie has given her some trouble. At least she does not feel her old self. We had quite a long chat. She told me she understood I had a very pleasant winter being under the protection of so many ladies. She tried to find out if I hear from any of them. I did not catch on worth a cent! I watched a very interesting operation, the removal of part of the lower jaw and the transplanting of a piece of sheep's jaw in its place. If it proves all right, I wonder if he will want to eat grass or hay!

I made the acquaintance of Miss Julia Cook. She resembles Dr. Mitchell[9] of Montreal. We were seated together. She is very clever, has been practising in a London hospital for 4 years. I learnt this from her: that *Rodent Ulcer never attacks the face below the level of the upper lip.* If I go to London, I am going to call on her.

One of the surgeons did a most splendid operation one day. He removed 21 inches of the intestine, sutured the ends together. The patient got quite well.

Some time ago a boy met with a severe burn, the Dr. grafted a piece of skin off a *pup* on him and it has healed nicely but the latest reports are that he trees every cat he sees and that he barks in his sleep! I shall let you know the results of the sheep jaw grafting.

Thus endeth the 38th chapter of "Chew the rag." This is by 11 pages the longest letter I ever wrote. Oh, the results came out in the paper this morning not in order of merit but in order of registration. I registered last.

Good bye.

P.S.   I had a letter from Dr. McGrath. He is practising in Chicago. He had *two* patients the first day.

(Rec. Oct. 30, 1889)

No. 6 Marchmont Crescent,
Edinburgh, Sept. 26, 1889

My dear Grace,

As I have a whiles intermission in the midst of a great hurry I hasten to reply to yours of the 2nd inst. which I rec. about 10 days ago. I was very glad to hear from you & to know you are enjoying life so thoroughly. Why, you have actually developed into a regular Dr. I was very much pleased to hear you have had such a profitable summer; in fact, I am delighted with you. Don't be the least afraid to tell me what you are doing, as I am the last one in the world to misconstrue anything you may tell me. I think we understand each other well enough to interchange medical experience; at least I venture to say you have already had a greater experience than any of the ladies in the final year, particularly in the treatment of your own sex. You say you feel ever so much older — that will never do. You must not take the sadness of life to heart too much: there is time enough for that in far off years to come.

I am awfully glad you told me about the receipt of a new nephew. I am also glad to know Mrs. Savage made a good recovery. Kindly remember me to her & tell her my best wish is that her darling baby boy may grow up to be a good and useful man.

No, you did not quite make me believe that I am in the possession of *Auburn locks* ha! ha! Why didn't you try and make me believe my eyes are *green* too. I quite agree with you that he is a fine fellow, altho, I have never met him, I know of him. He is not in the Western[10] dispensary now, is he? You might tell me about the row they had there. Just fancy putting a 2nd year student in a hospital as house Surgeon. You will wonder how I know all these things — don't you? Well, you know I am a *mind reader* & distance is no barrier; in fact I believe it makes it all the more *accurate*.

132 lbs. dear me, what have you been eating: & had you your summer dress on? Well you are a Lovely Fat-Porpoise in truth. Please excuse pet names for you know it would not be nice to be called an ordinary fat porpoise. What about "That Eyes" and "Those magnetism?" I suppose you can hardly see, and you know it is a physiological fact, the deeper nerves are situated the less sensitive they are. Well I think that is enough of *"Twaddle"* so I shall go on & write my letter.

Since writing you from Sanquhar I have had loads of work, & heaps of amusement. Oh, did you get the Scotch heather I sent you by parcel post, and there was a letter enclosed with it?

I had such a pleasant & profitable time at Sanquhar. I am happy to say I had no deaths to register during my stay there, altho, I thought one poor little congenitally syphilitic, rachitic youngster was going to bid goodbye to its unhappy parents, — but it didn't. After leaving Sanquhar I went to Dumfries, where I spent two days putting up in the King's Arm Hotel where Bobby Burns frequently spent his evenings. While there I saw something of Scotch hotel life. I had any amount of fun.

I was at a fine dog show in the Waverley Market the other evening. I saw all the different kinds of dogs. There were over 1000 altogether. I never saw a more howling exhibition!

I then went to Ecclefechan to visit my relations. I don't know when I enjoyed myself so much. My cousin, Dr. Cross, was in Edinburgh at the time so I telegraphed him to come down, & he did so. Well, we just broke loose & had fun to no end. We were at a Scotch dance one night — Great Scott! — those Scotch girls do dance, & everlastingly hug a fellow when it comes to the swinging. I fancied I had a pair of corsets on all the next day. We went to a country show where cattle, sheep, pigs, horses and people are exhibited. I was very much pleased with my relations, they were so kind and nice to us.

A drunk man ran into a short-sighted man on the street one day. The short-sighted man made profound apologies, telling him he was short-sighted. All right, old pard, said the drunk man, I forgive you and you are a gentleman for I have met a dozen short-sighted people on this street and none of them had the decency to apologize to me!

I saw Old Mortality that Scott writes about when in Dumfries. I was also up in a tower where every part of the city is reflected on a round table by means of glasses.

I was visiting my uncle at the same time another cousin from England, a young lady I had never met before, was there. Well, I haven't seen a prettier girl in Scotland. I believe if she hadn't been my cousin I would have been completely mashed. However, Cross fell under her charms. She isn't the least bit of a flirt, or she would be dangerous.

I met two very peculiar young ladies while there. They are in possession of a good deal of the mammon of unrighteousness. £10,000 or more & all they talk about is their ancient family. I horrified them when I told them that I was of a very ancient family too — in fact it dated away back before Christ. They didn't think there were any ancient families in America. Why, I said, "don't you know that's where Adam and Eve were born." Such information had the effect of making them at least somewhat natural, & encouraged them to talk about something more interesting than ancient families. My cousin, Miss Thompson, was tickled over the conversation as she had never seen them act so natural before.

Cross & I went to Carlisle in England to visit a cousin, Thos. Little. He was only married 4 or 5 months ago. He is a fine fellow, and his wife is just lovely. We then came back to Ecclefechan, visited Burnswick Hill where the ghosts & fairies play at night. It is the seat of an old Roman camp. The Roman walls are there still. To remember me that I too must die, I visited the graves of my forefathers. I found my great-grandfather & grandmother buried in Hoddom Church yard. Their monument is a funny one. It is as high as the church and the back of it looks like a stone chimney, the front is dressed stone with two round pillars. The Slab is built in near the top. My great-grandfather must have been a bit of a blarney, for, he had this inscription put on to his wife: —

"She was a virtuous wife
A loving mother
And one esteemed
By all who knew her."

And, to be short to her praise
she was the wife Solomon speaks
of in XXXI Chapt. Proverbs–10
verse to the end.

She died 1779.

While in Carlisle we went thru the Castle. We were in the dungeons. In one of them 50 men died in one night, in another 30 died in one night. The chains were there that they were bound with. Oh! it was beautifully horrible. In another dungeon Mary Queen of Scots was kept for some few weeks. Cross got a piece of a *match* that she used to light her cigarette *with*. I don't swear to the truth of his statement, but he says so & I am almost inclined to believe him altho history don't mention it. After having a whole week of enjoyment we returned to Edinburgh to resume work. Later news: Now, this is an awful secret, & if any person is in the room when you come to it just wait until they go out, & turn down the gas for fear some person is looking in at the window. Those young ladies we met, on several occasions, *told my* cousin, that *we, Cross* and *I,* are the *finest* young men they ever *met,* & that they would go to America if all the men there were like us. Cheers! Oh! how we did swallow the contents of that letter & how big we felt; for, some of those young damsels have travelled a good deal. Cross is beginning to think that "He's the man with the mashing eye" — that's English, quite English, you know! Oh yes, to use a theatrical expression they thought us "Devilish clever." I heard that at "My Brother's Sister," Minnie Palmer the American actress being the principal figure. Go & hear her if you have an opportunity.

No, electricity is used very little in the treatment of tumors. So far the results have not been satisfactory, in abdominal tumors. John Duncan, Surgeon to the Infirmary, has had excellent results with electricity in the treatment of Goitre, Subcutaneous Nervi, Cirsoid Aneurism and other Aneurisms. He uses needles insulated with vulcanite to within ½ in. from point. He thrusts the needles into the tumor, then attaches the battery and lets it run for ½ hour, moving the needles frequently. The needles are withdrawn slowly so as to coagulate the blood, and prevent bleeding. I have seen him treat quite a number in this way with the best results. Electricity is also used here in the treatment of tumors at the Pylorus. A hollow tube is passed into the stomach, then a wire with a copper point is passed through the tube to within an ⅛ in. from the end. The current is transmitted to the tumor through the fluids in the stomach. The other pole is placed on the outside over the seat of the tumor. The stomach should be carefully washed out first. I wonder how this would work on Mr. Allen at 40 Stewart St. [11]

Since I returned I have been taking a special course on practical Gynaecology four days in the week. There are only four in the class. Some days we have 20 patients. I have assisted with some very fine operations. I expect the Dr. will do two Laparotomies tomorrow. I am also taking a course on diseases of children, & also giving a good deal of attention to the eye.

Lacerations of the cervix are not treated by suturing now, even Emmet has practically given it up. Hot water applications and caustics and carbolic acid are used.

All solutions applied to the nostril should be mixed with common salt as it prevents irritation. A solution of salt applied to nostril will often stop sneezing when other things fail. Of course $AgNO_3$ would be an exception to the above rule.

I am only going to have the benefit of a little over a week of the post-graduate course. It lasts three weeks.

Well Grace, I have bought my ticket for Australia. I sail from Southampton per S.S. *Kaiser Wilhelm II*. It is a new vessel built by the North German Lloyd Coy. She made her maiden trip this month to New York & proved herself to be a pretty fast boat. I sail either on the 5 or 6th October so I hope to be in Australia by 10 of November if nothing happens. I hope to reach there in time to wish you a Merry Xmas and a Happy New Year.

I leave here for London either on Saturday evening or Monday, as I want to spend a few days with Cross, & I have some friends to visit also.

I would love so much to take the trip via Montreal, Toronto and Barrie, but I cannot do it. I would like so much to have a big long talk with you for I have so much to tell you; but I must not think of it as it only makes me feel uneasy. I wonder if I shall enjoy this winter as much as I did last. I did enjoy your company so much. You see old days have their charm and you know there are some feelings you cannot put into words or writing because some day they might look beautifully silly. Well, after all it is just a question whether our weaknesses or our strengths give us most pleasure; however, I shall not attempt to discuss this question here.

I am looking forward with a great deal of pleasure to meeting my brother in Australia. I have not seen him for two years. We spent a month together in Hamilton before he left, & I tell you we had a pleasant time of it. We can chum it together nicely. I have had four letters from him since I came here. He is getting along splendidly and has made a great many friends, particularly Drs. He has made the acquaintance & friendship of the belle of Adelaide. This young lady, and her brother, are going to meet me at the wharf when the boat calls. I think the boat remains there some 5 or 6 hours so I shall have a little opportunity of seeing what she is like.

I go as far as Melbourne where I expect to meet my brother. He wants me to take three weeks' holidays & he will show me the best parts of Australia. I do not know where in that part of the world I shall settle. If in a city it will either be Sydney or Melbourne. I have been offered a position to *lecture* in a college out there, but it is an Agricultural College, & that don't suit me. It would be on Physiology, Hygiene and some such stuff. I want to get settled in practice as soon as possible. The Mayor's son of the city of Melbourne is president of a lodge there and he has offered to give me the Surgery and Drship. of the lodge which would be worth $800 a year, and besides he will introduce me to the best families and do all he can for me. He is a great friend of my brother & is anxious that I should come out as soon as possible. This lodge has a Dr. at present but he is drunk half the time and therefore they are tired of him.

Robertson, the Australian, called me a few evenings ago and had me to a trained horse show in one of the theatres.

There is a Dr. in Sydney has a practice worth $35,000 a year and he wants an assistant or a partner & is anxious to see me. He has an assistant at present but he is no good. This Dr. is a great friend of *Jim's,* my brother. Jim has found a good opening in the country where a man can do well but will have hard work. I would like a country practice for a year. There is no place where a man gets such schooling as in the country. There you have to be thoroughly self-reliant and that is a training every man requires.

Do you know I really feel anxious at times and wonder how I shall get along. I don't feel the least discommoded to take another Dr.'s practice but it's different when you have to start for yourself. I shall just go ahead and treat what few patients I may get as scientifically as I know how and if they don't get better, science is to blame not me. Rather a nice way of flattering oneself, isn't it?

It is a very easy matter to cover up any mistakes in practice of medicine, but it can't be so easily done in surgery.

That was a sad suicide in Dominion Square & such a tragic history in connection with it. You would hardly expect such an affair to end up in Montreal. [12]

Now, Grace, as you are attending the Infirmary, I shall give you a page from my note book which you may find of a little service to you.

Lecture on Exam. of Urine:
1.   Always proceed to exam in a methodical manner.
2.   If possible note the quantity.
3.   Note the colour.
a)   Light = Diabetes, Diluted, Hysteria, Granular Kidney, etc.
b)   Dark = Concentrated, medicines, Fevers, acute Bright, cirrhosis of Liver, Severe Hemorrhage, etc.
c)   Froth = may have albumin or bile.
d)   Little fine scratches on the glass points to Oxolate of Lime.
e)   Flies gathering around the glass points to diabetes.
4.   Smell may be sweet or ammoniacal.
5.   Reaction = normal acid.
6.   Sp[ecific] gravity.
a)   low — diluted or albumin

b)   high — concentrated or *Sugar* or it has been doctored by the patient so as to be admitted into hospital. This is often tried in Edinburgh.

7.   Test for *Albumin first* — Hint — HNO_3, picric acid, etc.

8.   Sugar no less than six tests.

9.   Blood liq. pot, gives a dark app. Tinct. + Boric ether gives a beautiful blue.

10.   Bile add H_2SO_4 plus cane sugar gives a cherry red.

The reason I give you the above is that ½ the clinical exam in the hospital consists of the above. Students are frequently *ploughed* (a new expression) by going and testing for albumin first thing. You will have ample opportunity to carry out the tests and you will be agreeably surprised to find that you become quite an expert in a few days. Through the kindness of one of the House Surgeons, Dr. Abernathy, I mastered that part of the clinical work in three hours. For the tests refer to Roberts or any Practice of Medicine. You will find this of use to you in your exam in physiology next spring both in the College & Council. [13]

I shall now try and give you a diagram of two new bandages I learned to do since I came here. Divergent and Convergent spica. They allow the free motion of the knee and they maintain equal pressure. Useful in House Maid's Knee, which you will often be consulted about. I have just tried to give you an idea by sketching but it is a poor attempt:

No. 1 is the convergent spica of the knee. They all cross behind the knee. Begin at 1 by taking a turn around the leg above the knee, then the 2nd turn is around the leg below the knee. Continue this overlapping the bandage ⅔ until you meet in the centre over the knee cap where the full width of the bandage is shown at fig. 8.

No. 2 = Divergent bandgage — Begin at 1 by taking two turns around the knee cap then let the 2nd turn go up a little and the third below a little, showing the least little bit of the first turn. You finish by showing the full width of the bandage above and below the knee.

I want you to tell me if you succeed in understanding this bandage for it is a good one and I want you to introduce it in Kingston, as none of us ever saw it there.

I shall mail you a matrimonial paper just to let you see the *golden* opportunities a young man, particularly a middle aged man, has. I have no time to bother with such things or I would write some of them just to see how they would perform.

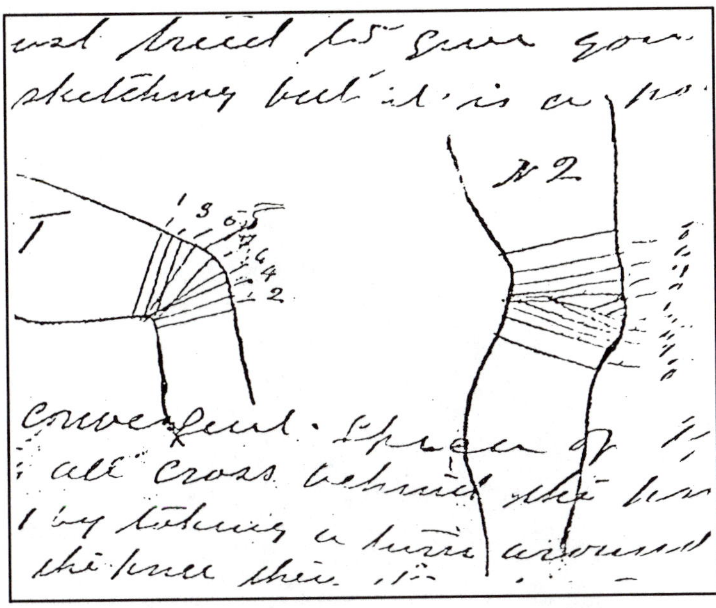

"Useful in House Maid's Knee. . . . I have just tried to give you an idea by sketching but it is a poor attempt"

I shall be busy for the next day or two packing up my things, a job I much dislike. I have an awful lot of stuff as I have invested in a lot of books, clothes, etc. I even became extravagant enough to buy a full dress suit of the best quality. I shall be real glad when I get settled for I am getting tired of knocking about so much.

I trust you and your friend will get suitable rooms in Kingston. If you get as comfortable lodgings as I have, you will be happy. There are very few good places in Kingston.

You must call and see little Miss Fair. She is becoming more interesting every day, so I heard.

If you meet a Mr. McLennon, a 3rd year M.D. student, I think you will find him rather nice. He was over here this summer. I fancy Ned Ryan will be back in college this winter. He is a true fellow. I had a letter from

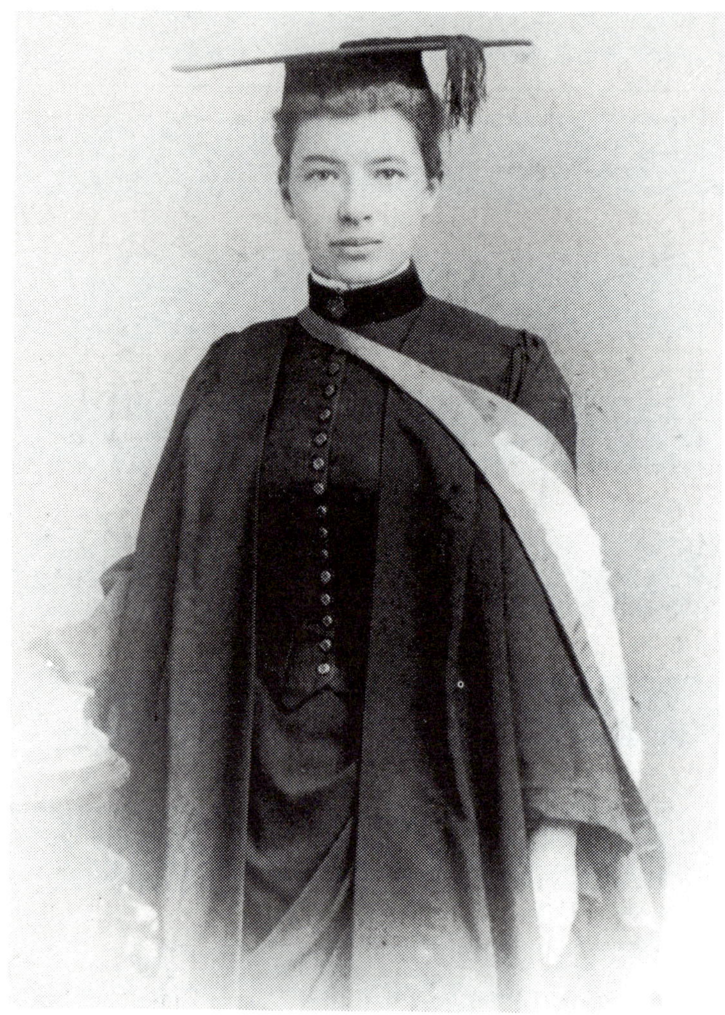

"I like that photo with the cap and gown"

Dean McGrath. He is doing nicely in Chicago. He has a telephone in his office. I expect to hear from Jack (Dr. Roberston) next mail.

Now when you get settled nicely in Kingston write me and tell me all the news. Find out when the mail leaves Frisco so your letter won't lie there a month. If you write me shortly after you go to Kingston the letter will be waiting me in Melbourne for it will take me six weeks to reach there. Address me to:

Bourke St. East P.O.
Melbourne, Australia

Oh say, when you get any cabinet photos taken I want you to give me one, won't you? I like that photo with the cap and gown but as you only have the one I won't ask it. You know that little gem is not a good photo of you.

You will have quite a hard winter's work but one good thing, you have no chemistry to bother with.

It will be awfully hot in Australia. I shall just reach there about the beginning of summer. I shall be sure to melt for I am terribly fat.

My cousin, Dr. Cross,[14] will be in Montreal for a few days on his way home. He will be there about Xmas. Do you mind if he calls on you? He is jolly and very outspoken. It is worth 50 cts. to hear him laugh a good laugh. He knows of you for his sister's friend met Shuttleworth who gave her a glowing account about you and of course I told him enough to make him anxious to see you.

Now, Grace, don't be praying for me to be seasick for I shall have enough of inconvenience from the heat without the addition of any other troubles. I must bid you goodbye and remember your letters will always be welcomed with a warm heart. Kindly remember me to your mother and sister.

I remain
Your sincere friend
William C. Little

P.S.   I am afraid of these skinny letter envelopes breaking loose and spilling the contents. If one is strong, two must be much stronger.

I shall mail you one of Byron Bromwell's clinics. He publishes some of the best cases every month. You can see what a treat students get at some of the clinics. I wish Chown,[15] your lovely old "Snipe," would make an endeavour to give something like them.

Medical conundrum: In Pseudo-hypertropic paralysis the boys are always affected and how is it that it can always be traced back to the mother. Ans: The boys all die, therefore there are no fathers to trace it to! Ask the final ladies this conundrum.

(Rec. Dec. 28, 1889
Montreal. Xmas holidays)

Bourke St. East P.O
Melbourne, Nov. 25, 1889

My dear Grace,

Here I am alive & kicking, in the very best of health & spirits, but awfully easily tired out when I take a long or short walk. A very funny thing I experienced when I landed was that I became almost sick. I imagined the streets and ground, houses & everything were rolling about. Just fancy, I spent 7 Sundays on the sea.

Before going any further I must thank you for writing me so promptly for, to my great delight, your letter was waiting me in Melbourne. It was just like meeting your best friend in a foreign land. Your letter seemed to shake hands with me & say I am so glad to welcome you to a new country. It made me feel as if I were only a few miles from home. You just hardly understand what a pleasure it gave me.

Dear me, you won't be a bit interested in what I have to tell you for it is all ship (not shop).

After leaving my cousin Dr. Cross in London I came to Southampton, remained there one night & embarked for here next morning before I had time to get my breakfast. The *Kaiser Wilhelm II* is the finest boat I ever saw; in fact, she is the finest Eastern vessel afloat. We had a few storms but nothing serious, just enough to relieve the monotony of the voyage.

We stopped two days at Genoa, which gave me ample time to visit the places of interest & gain a little knowledge of how Italians live. Genoa is a very pretty place. Her churches & cathedrals are grand beyond my ability to describe. I was through the art galleries, universities, theatres, cemeteries, etc. While there the Italian fleet came in. I saw some 17 gun boats. Prince Henry of Prussia was there & visited the *Kaiser Wilhelm II.* I was just taken with him, he was so unassuming. There is a quiet manliness about him that I liked.

German boats are all very well but German people, cooks, stewards, captain & all, I simply detest. Germans seem to be clothed with skin 40 feet thick and that super-saturated with grease. Growling is one of the chief amusements on a long sea voyage & so we all *growled* and *growled.*[16] Oh, by the way, you lived in Germany for some time. Well, did they serve you with meat, gravy, potatoes, cabbage, prunes and rice all on one plate at the same time? How it did amuse me to see the hoggish dishes they put down for us to eat.

I just look on Germans as slop buckets into which may be thrown anything you choose. Enough of that.

The Mediterranean Sea was calm nearly all the way, the climate simply delightful, just like 2000 miles of love — one pleasant dream. That looks almost like poetry but it isn't for at present my poetical inclinations are at a low ebb. I am not myself yet — the continual change — the great change has produced a kind of shock in which poetry does not form a part.

I visited Port Said for the 3rd time[17] and found it just as great a Hell hole as ever. I spent a good while in a gambling den watching men and women losing their money. It is really a pretty picture to watch a woman gambling. All the phases of character that are expressed in a few minutes, woman, angel, friend. Women are the best gamblers in the world and of course take more pleasure out of it.

We went through the Canal during the night. They use large electric reflectors on the bow of the boat which enables them to take ships through at night. The Canal is a dreary place. How sad I felt while going through part of the Canal early in the morning to see those poor camels carrying great heavy loads of sand on their backs at the places where the canal was being widened. The poor things would lie down to let the men fill the great large sacks with sand and the brutes had to carry it quite a distance from the boat before unloading.

Are you fond of oranges? If so, they can be bought in Port Said for 2d per dozen.

We remained for 36 hours at Suez. I never had such sport in my life as I had there. The town of Suez is about 2 ½ miles from the Port. Nine of us went ashore and engaged donkeys to take us up to the town. What comical men those donkey-men are! They call their donkeys after illustrious characters, for e.g.: "Gladstone," "Mrs. Maybrick," "Mary Anderson," "Two Lobely Black Eyes" & a "Devil to go." The last-mentioned I secured & I found him to be all that the name implies, for I won the race both going and coming. It was a terrible hot day & I was the only one [who] had the good sense to take an umbrella. You would have gone into fits if you had seen us. Imagine me starting out with my umbrella up & the donkey trotting along quietly, then we started to race, still the umbrella was up & I kept it up until I got near the town, when I closed it and used it to make the donkey go. Each donkey has a man to make it go and those poor beggars ran with us fully 10 miles. How they beg to go with you to earn a 6d. They say "Me good donkey-boy." Fancy a man bragging himself up to be a good donkey-boy. After we reached Suez we did up the town — when we landed in the town the nine of us set up such a war whoop that we frightened the natives. Next we got a new supply of donkeys & went out to the fresh water canal. I came in third last on this trip, but I got my "Devil to go" to take me back to the port & won the race twice out of three, which was not so bad.

The Red Sea was very hot, not a breath of air. After we got into the Arabian sea the weather was lovely. The boat stopped 48 hrs. at Colombo, Ceylon — dear old Colombo! the place where I went to seek my fortune & didn't find it. I met some familiar faces at the British India Hotel. It seems to be my fate to visit every place twice. (I wonder if I shall visit Australia twice.) While at Colombo, 4 of us hired a cab and drove some 8 miles up the country to a Buddhist Temple. What a delightful drive through the avenues of palm and coconut trees all laden with bananas and nuts. I am in love with Ceylon, all mashed, & so would you if you were there awhile. While at the Buddhist temple I bought two little Gods, offerings to his Godship Buddha, one of which I enclose to you. It is pure silver. You can keep the little baboon in your pocketbook to keep ghosts away or anything else you like. I think it would look better if it were dressed up a little, but I shall leave that for your dainty fingers to do.

We stopped a short time in Adelaide, long enough for me to make a few calls and here I must say I have never [met] finer people than the Australians. I felt at home immediately. The people are very kind and friendly. By the way, my friend Billy whom you have heard me speak about — the fellow that was with me in Quebec — met me at Adelaide. He is the best-hearted soul in the world. Poor Billy, he travels around a great deal, meets many young ladies & he is so kindhearted he has to make love to them but he does not stop there for he engages himself to them. He is at present engaged to six. "Damn it" he says, "what am I to do — I can't marry them all?" You could not meet a more natural and outspoken fellow. He is staying here with my brother & I. [sic.] We have any amt. of fun. He is really the funniest man I ever knew. All the girls like him. He is all mashed on a Jewess, very wealthy, & he is going to propose tonight. My brother was preparing a few practical sentences for his use. This young lady's brother is an M.P. & he has been very kind to me. I think it is really too bad for Billy to go on like that but he won't listen to reason, he simply says he is

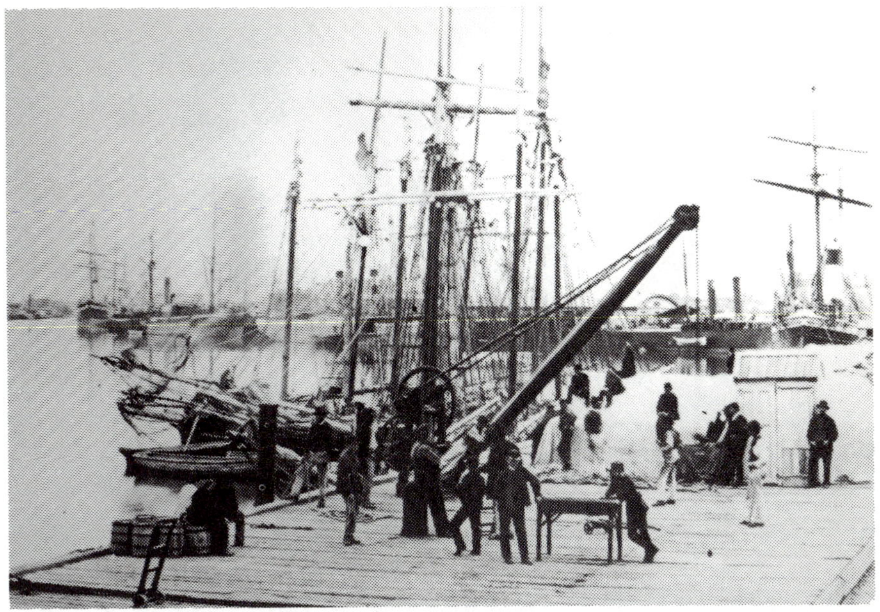

The harbour at Melbourne circa 1890

in love & he is going to propose & propose he will. You will think him crazy but he isn't. He has a government position & an easy life. I shall tell you more of this interesting character at another time.

My brother met me at the wharf in Melbourne, he is looking fine. How pleased I was to meet him. Shortly I came to the Osbourne House where I am now. He presented me with a solid gold chain worth about £12.[18] There is a beautiful green stone on it, on the stone there is a gold hand grasping a heart. I also got some other useful presents.

Well Grace, I really do not know yet where I shall locate. There are a number of country openings quite near my Cousin, Dr. Cross.[19] I am going tomorrow to have a look at them. I want to settle in a town but they are nearly as well filled as the towns at home. I have my mind set on a stall in one of the suburbs of Melbourne. The difficulty settling in the city is the very high rents & my want of capital. If I do go to the country it will only be to make enough money to start in a town or city. At present I cannot say what I shall do, but will be able to let you know by my next letter.

While in Genoa I noticed a scarf a great many of the ladies wore so I bought one for you. It may help to keep your throat warm. I am only sorry I could not get you a nicer one. I shall mail you it inside a newspaper

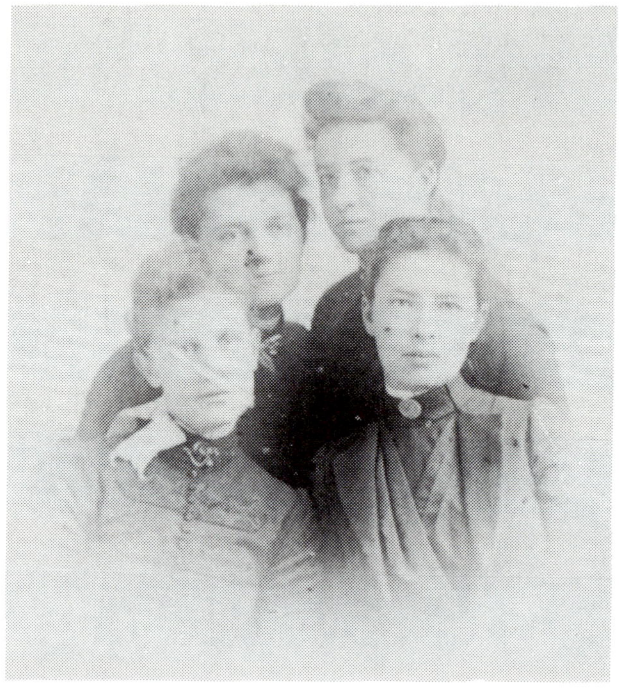

*"Kindly remember me to the Menagerie. Poor Miss Bennett's face in the picture
got scratched a little; the glass broke"*

so if the paper goes astray you will not get it. Whenever I mail you a newspaper
there will be something enclosed.

I hope your little Savage nephew is enjoying good health. I suppose
he will soon be getting teeth.

Why, you astonish me when you tell me what a specialist you have
become. You have got ahead of me altogether. I can hardly imagine the
jolly rosy-faced girl of last winter with all her treasures spread out on the
floor around her springing up & casting those things to the wind & in a
flash developing into a woman & a physician at the same time.

I am glad you have found comfortable quarters. I know the room
well. Yes, you have a hard winter's work before you, but you must not hurt
yourself trying to do too much.

Kindly remember me to the Menagerie.[20] Poor Miss Bennett's face
in the picture got scratched a little; the glass broke. Oh, a "hindoo" at Colombo wanted to buy that tie pin you gave me.

I shall write you next mail, by which time I shall have my thoughts collected & will give you a little Australian News. Glad you succeeded in getting a hospital change. My brother wishes me to wish you a pleasant Xmas & a happy New Year. He told me that he liked your photo. I must close by wishing you all the joys imaginable during Xmas vacation. You will be home when you see this.

Sincerely,
Your wandering friend,
W.C. Little

P.S. I feel so stupid that I can't write a letter home. I am only going to send some Xmas cards & a ¼ page letter. I have not time to read this letter over as the mail closes in a very short time. Dr. Duff is well & flourishing.

(Rec. Jan 29th, 1890)

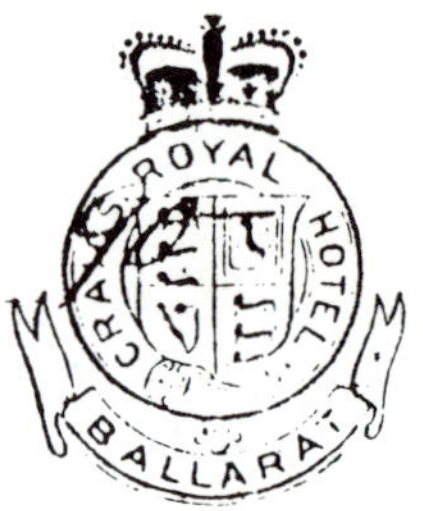

Craics Royal Hotel
Ballarat Dec 21st, 1889

My dear Grace

Just a few lines to wish you a very happy New Year and many happy returns on your birthday. [21] I have really forgotten the date of your birthday, but I know it is somewhere between now and spring. I know it came after the reunion last year.

I am in this beautiful town for the night — I am quite in love with it and would like to settle here, but a great many other Drs. were of the same feeling and therefore have left very *little* room for me. I am taking my cousins's, Dr. Cross, practice for a few weeks — not here but in Horsham. There is lots of work — a large practice and a hospital to look after. The fact of the matter is ever since I came out here I have simply been enjoying myself and have not until now felt anything like settling down. I have not decided where I shall settle yet. I am not going to be in a big hurry as I want to get acquainted with the people and know their ways and also become acquainted [with] Australian diseases by doing Locum Tenens work for a month or two. You see, if I make any mistakes I have not to live in the place and suffer the consequences. By the way, I ran across "The Devil's Due" by Grant Allen yesterday. I have read about 100 pages. It is very good so far. The "Hindoo" is just a little too clever at reading symptoms. Dr. Harry C. is a rare specimen; those lovely snakes and poisons in his laboratory are simply charming. How could the artist help falling in love? How true Olwen is to womankind longing to have 2 or 3 hearts to give around to soothe the troubled breasts of those who fell victim to her charms. So far *she* is a beautiful character. Why did you tell me to read this book? Was it because I remarked one day if Mr. so and so would die in the Hospital I would find out what was the matter with him? I wonder if it is not possible that such thoughts enter every Dr.'s head without him ever thinking what they mean. A good motto is the answer a Dr. in an Egyptian hospital gave Napoleon when he asked him, "Would it not be better to end the suffering soldiers' lives?" — "The physician's mission is to cure not to kill."

I had quite an experience the other day on a R.R. car. I got tired riding in the car, so I asked the engineer to let me ride with him. Great United States! — he did make that car go. I told him to tell me the most blood curdling things he could. So he said: "Do you see that curve ahead, the rails often spread and the engine is smashed to pieces" and he said pointing to a glass indicator, "That would burst at 150 lbs. steam and there are 145 on now." To tell you the truth I was glad to get off the blamed thing. I don't think I looked discommoded but I felt it.

I am just beginning to feel myself again. I felt regularly mixed up for a week or two after I landed. I could not think to write home so I got my brother to do it for me.

By the way I had a letter from my cousin, Dr. Cross of London, he is not going home for another 8 mos. or a year.

I mailed you some Melbourne views, a Sydney view and a birthday card. I also sent you a paper with a picture of native courtship in it: I hope you like them. The native way of courting is to hide somewhere until the object of his affections happens to pass by, the manly lover jumps out from amongst the bushes, knocks her down with a club & carries her off wholesale. How would you like that style of courtship?

I had a letter from Mr. Fair last mail, he said you had called at Allens. I fancy 40 Stewart St. is not quite so lively as last winter. Well, we had heaps of fun there. I just wish I could have some of the good old times over again.

Remember me to your sister Mrs. Savage. I suppose she never thinks of Lachute now since she found that wonderful baby. I hope the child is enjoying good health.

How is poor Mrs. Walker? I often feel sorry for her, she suffers so much and is so terribly sensitive. How is the *Porpoise, Hen* & *Whale.* I was asked today what fish I liked. I said the Porpoise by all means. The waiter said he did not know any fish of that name. Ask Miss Demerest if she likes my *system* any better this year than last. Great Scott, I did not think she heard me that night.

So Jack Shannon is engaged. Well, he will get a good deal of wealth with her. I never met her but have seen her. He will be related to Allens at 40 [Stewart St.]. Jack Duff has settled in a good district; 30 miles from a R.R. I may not settle for 2 or 3 months yet. I must close by wishing you every possible good and remaining your sincere friend.

Wm. C. Little

P.S. 1 — I hope you have quite recovered from your *cold,* if not go to bed and don't stir out until you get better. How does that advice catch you?

P.S. 2 — When I get better acquainted I shall tell you what I think of Australians. I cannot believe that this is Xmas, no snow — grain & fruits ripe — I feel lost almost.

P.S. 3 — Melbourne is a grand city. I would settle there only I would require £2000 to begin with, which I have not at present.

(Rec. Feb. 25, 1890, Kingston
Ans.)

Bourke St. East P.O.
Melbourne, Jan. 23, 1890

My dear Grace,

It is now 11 p.m. and I have been waiting all day until now for the weather to get a little cooler, but in vain have I waited, for to add to the heat, the gas is burning. Hot! Hot! hot! is no name for it. Make the O an E and the T an LL and it would give you some idea of what I am enduring. Just fancy 98 degrees in my room. I am dressed I shall not tell you how for fear you would be shocked.

In the first place I must tell you that I received your letters of Nov. 11 and Dec. 5 all right but both at the same time. To say your letters were interesting would not do them justice. They were splendid, delightful, a regular treat. I read and reread them. I would much rather answer them in person than attempt to give you as good in return. My imagination stretched far enough to see you pillowed up in bed as you wrote. I hope you have got over that cold; it is terrible to have it hanging on so long. Why does the dear old "Snipe" not get you cured up? I am sure I would have had you better by this time. Remember those colds are not to be fooled with, they should be sat on at their very first appearance.

When I rec. your letters I was going down to a drug store. I had to wait some little time so began reading the first one. The first thing I knew, some who were in the store were staring at me. I unconsciously had been laughing over Miss H. knowing what I wanted the splints for. Do you know I suspected as much. Miss H. cannot be fooled very easily, still she went to Napanee! I am so sorry you did not succeed in getting a good cast. Well, I sincerely thank you for the attempt. We will just have to "Learn to labor and to wait" — you to labor and I to wait.

The Xmas number of the *Star* is quite good and was much admired by quite a number of Australians. It was very kind of you to send it. I am going to have some of the pictures framed and hung up in my office, which office I expect to exist in some 4 or 5 more days.

I hope to begin practice for myself this week in a little town about 190 miles from Melbourne and 40 miles from my Cousin, Dr. Cross. My reasons for going there are that I have made a slight name there already

Dr. Little, assisted by Dr. Young, performed a successful operation at the Horsham hospital on Sunday. It was a case of empyema—a large amount of pus having collected in a cavity in the chest, and fully a gallon of liquid was drawn out. The patient, a Chinaman named Charles Ah Wong, is progressing favorably.

and I have been asked by the most influential people in the town to go there. While taking my cousin's practice, which I mentioned in my Ballarat letter, I had some interesting surgical cases. I had one case of Empyema which I tapped on Sunday and took 5 or 6 pints of pus; the following Sunday I operated on him and took out 7 pints. I cut down between the ribs and put in a drainage tube. The case is doing well. By some means, I think through the papers a young man about 30 miles from there heard of me, and came to be examined. He had been treated by another Dr. I found one side of the chest dull, enlarged, the heart displaced to the left. I tried succussion, i.e., shaking him — the first time I ever tried it; and distinctly heard the fluid rattling in his chest. I stuck a trocar in between the 6 and 7 ribs, and drew off 3 pints of fluid. These were two rare cases and how they happened to fall into my hands is rather strange and yet very fortunate for me. I had no less than 17 cases of typhoid fever.

I am going to like practice very much. In the town I am going to the fees are good, nothing under 10/6 ($2.60). That is a little better than Canada. A medical man is looked up to much more than at home. The Dr. ranks first here or equal and the lawyer 3rd.

You will want to know if I like the country, well, I can hardly say yet. I am not a bit in love with Australia. There is a decided want of moral tone everywhere. Drinking and its accompanying evils are found in all parts. There is an awful lot of looseness, free and easy style amongst both sexes. This is too bad. How few really have the strength to master a great temptation. There are forces too strong for some men and they yield simply because they cannot help it. Drink seems to be the great temptation here. The climate is such that people have to drink something and soft drinks are not always chosen, as may be noticed on the streets every night. The water is not good and the report that typhoid germs are in it give sufficient excuse for not drinking it.[22] I wonder if Lizabeth in "Devil's Due" could see the germs of Typhoid as well as the cholera germs.

That novel is certainly interesting, but I could scarcely believe that Dr. Chechil would try to poison his lovely little wife. No, No, that was over drawn. Miss Moyne I disliked very much. On her first appearance she was positively rude to the Dr.'s wife. She was not a lover of Mrs. Grundy, although I think Mrs. Grundy holds her place in moral reforms or the prevention of the necessity of reforms.

Have you read "The Continent of America" by Max O'Neil. It is quite good. Continue to inform me of your reading outside of Anatomy as it may stimulate me to the perusal of works I know nothing of.

So you think of trying for the scholarship. Well, you have my best wishes for your success. I am satisfied you will not have the least difficulty in winning it. I will bet on you, and Miss Henderson 2nd. Remember, don't go and hurt yourself for the sake of a paltry scholarship.

Oh, I received a very nice letter from Edinburgh stating that I have been made a Fellow of the Obstetrical Society. I am quite pleased for every Dr. can't get that. I made a good friend of the Secretary of the Society and assisted him in quite a number of operations and it was he that proposed me. You can never get that because you can never be a Fellow! Isn't that a pity? I don't think so.

Well, Grace, I have not had the pleasure of meeting a *"Maori"* yet — I don't know when I shall. I suppose when I do meet her I will knock her down with a club and run off with her. What a jolly way to make love, to become a wife unconsciously or nearly so must save a woman's feelings very much, and besides it saves minister's fees, etc.

I have only seen one native. They are becoming very scarce. About the only use they are put to is to hunt the woods for lost children. They are credited with being able to smell tracks like a dog even days after a person has walked over the ground. They are called the "Black trackers."

Your letter made me feel lonesome when you spoke about going home at Xmas. You would have such a jolly time, how I wish I could have dropped down in Montreal for a few days, but why talk about impossibilities.

I went out in the garden and had a good feed of ripe strawberries. I was at a nice ball at the Agricultural College on the 3rd inst. I enjoyed myself very much as I was well acquainted with Prof. Brown and family in Guelph.[23]

I was surprised to hear that Ned Ryan has started practice in Kingston. I cannot see for the life of me how all the Drs. make a living. He may do pretty well there but I fear not.

Where are you going to start practice when you get through? I think you had better come out here and settle near me and then we could consult together. How funny than would be. I am afraid we would have more consultations that would be good for the patients, still the old proverb says "In the multitude of consultations there is safety." I won't take my oath that that is right, but is as nearly so as I can remember. Do you remember our first consultation down in the little house below the hospital? I was amused at watching you give the hypodermic injection. I saw then that you had the material to make a pretty good Dr. and I am sure you will be if you wish. You will remember my advice not to spoil yourself as a woman to become a Dr. for I think you will always be admired more as the former than the latter.

I often think of the good talks we had at 40 [Stewart St.] and wish I could have some of them over again. You know it is so much easier to talk than to write. The old custom I have not forgot and the glass of water, but then you know you must not let fingers touch for it would be very naughty and Miss H. would be shocked. I have often been sorry for being so unkind sometimes, but you know nature is a peculiar thing and will assert itself in very variable ways without our knowing just exactly why.

So Miss Herd is not married yet. I wonder whose fault it is. She is naturally fickle — out of sight, out of mind, but that is not strange for women are generally credited with that failing. I am quite satisfied the reports that were floating around last winter were untrue.

I have been busy the past few days buying things to begin housekeeping. I feel as green as green can be about such things. I do not know whether I shall take my meals in a hotel or get some woman on the shady side of 40 to keep house for me. I believe the latter would be the better plan. I am getting a horse & buggie so am looking forward to doing a good deal of driving, a thing I always enjoy.

I am sorry I cannot write better. Practically, the science of penmanship is no easy task, particularly if you have an hereditary predisposition to write badly, as I have. I discovered this failing amongst my friends in Scotland, the boys only being affected. I fancy I am too old to improve now.

It is growing late or early so I must close. The palmistry poetry was quite good. Yes, your fortune will come true if you can only understand it. I would willingly exchange fortunes with you but I won't say what fortune

---

I mean. I really think you should have that Palmistry framed as a puzzle for I don't think you understand it and I'm sure I don't. It will be as good as pigs in clover.

Out at one of the suburbs, St. Kilda Beach, a fine porpoise was seen last week and the papers made a great talk about it.

It would be such great fun if you would come jumping up here sometime. Let me know and I shall be there to pull you out. You had better bring the whale and hen with you for company and if you get hungry the whale and porpoise could eat the hen. A little nonsense now and then, you know.

My brother is enjoying good health and doing very well. He says he will with the greatest of pleasure call on you when he goes back. I told him I would not give your address. A peculiar thing is whatever girl I like he likes, and vice versa.

I am going to get some *Illustrated London News* to put on my office table for patients to look over when they have to wait.

In the course of your studies and lectures if you come across anything new just mention it for my benefit.

Oh, did you get a copy of one of Byron Bromwell's clinics I sent you? They are good and I advise you to subscribe for them, they are so interesting. I fancy they can be got in some of the medical bookstores. They can be got here.

In my next letter I shall tell you all about my housekeeping and practice. Give my kind regards to the Menagerie. I suppose Mrs. Walker never thinks of me now. Glad to see in the medical journal that Miss Demerest passed Council.

"Well, supposing" — do you ever say that now?

Now, good-bye and be good, and remember I am always delighted to hear from you.

Your sincere — Wm. C. Little

P.S. 1. I was in a Chinese den not long ago and smoked two pipes of opium. I felt glorious. I shall not try it again.
P.S. 2. The temp. in the sun today was 150.

(Rec. March 22, 1890
Ans. Kingston——)

Warracknabeal,
Victoria,
Australia.
Feb. 16, 1890

My dear Grace,

I have just come in from visiting a friend's place a short distance out of town. I am feeling pretty full, not in the sense we understand it in Canada, but in its literal sense for I have been eating all kinds of fruit — pears, peaches, pomegranates, grapes, figs, oranges and mulberries, all of which grew in the garden. The chief of the police and his wife just called to pay me a friendly visit. Nothing like keeping on the good side of those fellows, you know. P.M.'s have to be done up here occasionally for which the Dr. rec. good remuneration.

Well, here I am in *my own* surgery, feeling as comfortable and happy as possible. I have rented a very nice house with a beautiful garden in front and grape vines growing up on front of the veranda. The house is small, only 4 rooms, but I am having a kitchen and servant's bedroom put up. The surgery is not so large as I would like it, but it is comfortable. It has a cosy little fireplace in it which I like very much, especially when I indulge in smoking, which I have not given up yet. I am going to use one room as a waiting room, 1 as a surgery, 1 as a bedroom and the other for a dining room so that I shall occupy all the house.

I bought a buggie last week for $250, it cost six months ago $400. I consider I have the finest buggie in a radius of 50 miles. It has a fine leather top to keep both sun and rain off. I am going to buy a pair of horses shortly. In the meantime I hire when I want them. I shall keep a groom to look after the horses, cut wood, fix up the garden and *black boots*. I may say I have not blacked my shoes since I left Canada. I have been here nearly 3 weeks, during which time I have been very busy getting things fixed up. Oh how green I feel about buying the necessary things to start house-keeping. At last I got one good lady to make me out a list of what things I would require — saucepans, etc. which will save me a host of annoyance.

I have done a little in practice, but it is increasing every day, people are only beginning to find out I am here.

Shortly after I came here a man came pounding at the hotel and shouting for the new Dr. I drove 20 miles out in the country to see the patient. It was a case of premature labor, the child having been dead for about 3 or 4 weeks. The woman had nearly bled to death. I had to remove the child in pieces, which took me some 35 minutes. The woman is making a good recovery and a good advertisement for me. I only went to her once and for which I shall charge $75. A few nights afterwards I was called to a confinement case; when I arrived I found the patient in hysterical convulsions. As it was in the 2nd stage I delivered with forceps. This patient made a good recovery and for which I charge $30. I charge 7 shillings 6 pence a mile to go out in the country so that I do not mind going 20 or 40 miles. I was called 12 miles last week to see a Scotch lady. She sent for me because she heard I studied in Edinburgh.

I am beginning to feel quite at home now and am liking the country better all the time. The hot weather is over and the climate is just delightful. I think with a reasonable amount of sickness and success in treating it I shall do very well here.

The country is so different from Canada. There is no scenery at all in this part. It is a Dutch paradise — it is one continuous plain. You could not find a hill 5 ft. high.

There is a nice little river close by from which the town gets its water supply. I forgot to say I have a comfortable bath room in the house which I enjoy very much every morning.

I have engaged a woman to keep house for me. I have not seen her so I am taking her on speculation. She has to come all the way from Tasmania. "What a funny thing to do," I hear you say. Well, she has been very highly recommended by her cousin and his wife, and this lady and gentleman I consider are about as nice people as are in this place. This woman has been a school teacher in her time and at present is keeping house for her brothers which she finds is too hard work. She has reached the sensible age of 36, which is an important thing for you know people will talk and this place is the essence of gossip. Mrs. Grundy flourishes here like a big sun flower.

There is very little society here that I shall care about, so I suppose I shall have to live on the past and hope for the future.

You can scarcely form any idea of what this country is like. The first few weeks I was in it I swore I would leave it, never to return, but after a time I found myself becoming adapted to the change and now I believe I like it as well as Canada. I could drive hundreds of miles here without

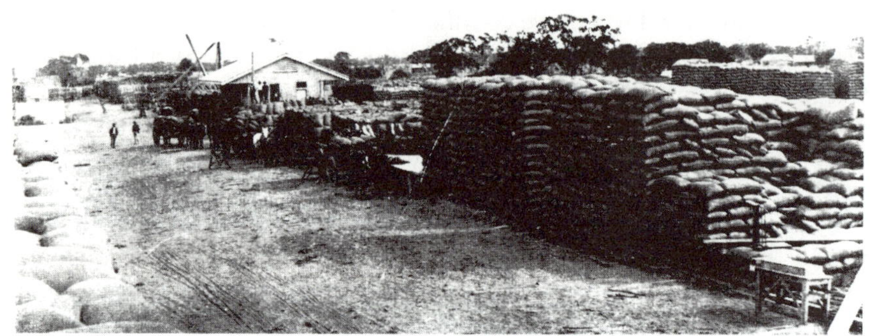

"The grain is all sold in 4 bush. bags and these bags are piled up 20-25 ft. high at the station. . . . There are no barns to put the grain in"

the least variation in the ground, not the sign of a hill. Oh, how flat, you say. So do I.

This is a farming town and it would astonish you to see the crude looking farmers as they come in with their loads of grain. An average load of grain in Canada is 50–75 bushels, here 300–400 is a load and it is drawn by 8 yoke of oxen or nearly as many horses. There will be about 1,500,000 bushels of wheat come into this town. The grain is all sold in 4 bush. bags and these bags are all piled up 20–25 ft. high at the station. The farmers do not cut the grain as in Canada, they have machines which pull the heads off and thresh it at the same time. The grain is cleaned in the field, put into bags and stacked up. There are no barns to put the grain in.

There is very little buggie driving done here, all horse-back riding. Every man, woman and child can ride on horseback. It is a very pretty sight to see a doz. horsemen come into the town together on fiery steeds. I have done a little riding but find it tires me out very quickly. I am glad I learned to ride when I was a kid. In fact I began to ride horses when I was 5 years old. A man asked me to try his horse the other day and I could see by the sardonic grin on his face he thought I could not ride. I jumped on his horse and gave it a good warming and then told the man his horse was a poor saddle beast.

I have found out what a pickaninny means. It is the Australian native word for a young baby, so please don't call poor Holdcroft that anymore.

I am thinking of getting a ½ caste for a groom as they are good horse men and as good as a dog to find the roads. I could drive you 10 miles out of town and you could never find your way back, the roads are mixed up so. I had such a charming drive a few evenings ago in the moonlight. I felt my whole being thrilled. I never remember seeing a finer evening. My brother is quite in love with this country. At present he is in Sydney. I think he has about the happiest and easy life one could wish for.

I received 4 letters from home yesterday, telling me all about the fun they had at Xmas. It made me feel a little bit sad or homesick — a feeling I cannot describe. In the letter from home to make me feel sure they were in good health my 4 sisters got weighed and sent me the weights which were: 113, 134, 152, *162*. What a weight of sisters I have, & just fancy when I was at home I could pile them all up in a heap, much to their annoyance.

I was living in anticipation of rec. a letter from you this mail to tell me all about your Xmas enjoyments, but it did not come. Your last two letters were so good that I shall just have to content myself until the next mail comes in, which will be in a long month.

What are you going to do this summer? If you have nothing special on I shall make you a *grand* offer to come here and attend the sick babies and dispense medicine, for which I will pay you $100 cash, board and washing and a pair of horses either to drive or ride when you like. I shall also grind you on Practice and Surgery to your heart's content. Now I really think this is a more liberal offer than the Napanee contract. What do you think?

There is nothing like having lots of good openings. Probably you can do much better in Montreal, still it is something to say you refused so and so. This letter will go to Montreal and be forwarded to you at Kingston so you can tell the Menagerie that you rec. a letter from Montreal with the above offer. See if Miss Henderson will catch on to it as well as she did the splints. If I only had the cast I would have it on the mantel-piece. I must tell you I have not seen a better model since I left Lachute. I wish I could spend a few days in Lachute this spring. Do you remember the race we had down the rapids? I didn't think you could run so fast.

So you think you will finish in Bishop's, Montreal. I think I would not if I were you, for you know Bishop's College has a poor standing compared with Queen's, and it is possible the day may come when Bishop's will be a thing of the past, which Queen's will never be.[24] Queen's is fast becoming a first-class university, 2nd to none. No doubt the hospital advantages in Montreal are much greater, but if you spend the summer months in hospital work you don't require much in the winter. However, you know what is best for yourself.

Poor girl, I suppose you are working night and day with a face as long as your arm as you plod over Anatomy, Physiology, Histology, Materia

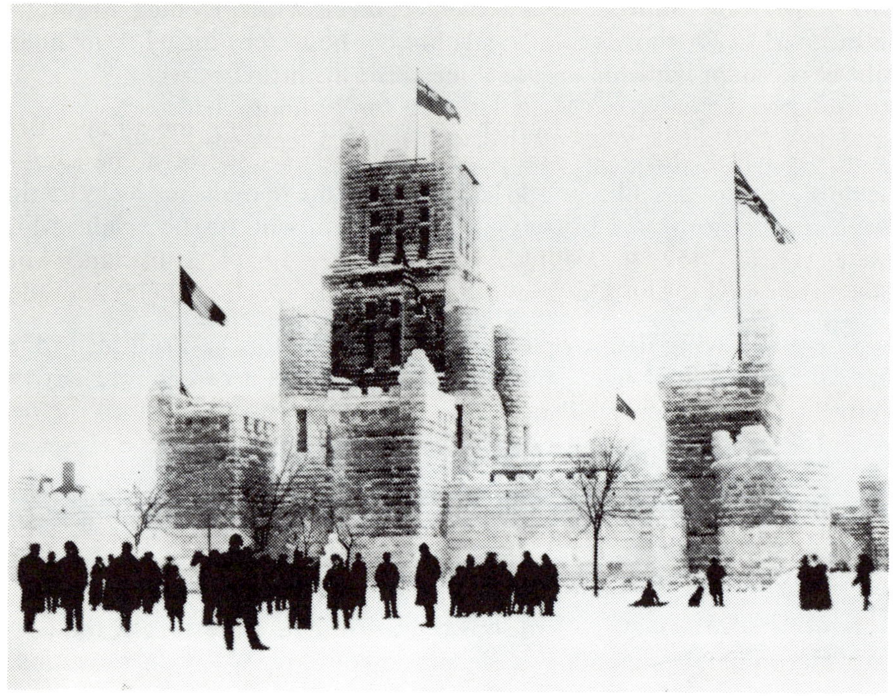

"You remember the picture of the ice palace you gave me, well I have it over the mantle-piece. It is much admired by all who see it"

Medica, etc. and then the dread Council to face. I will just give you a point when you go up for your oral at the council. I don't know whether you know that you can look very pleasant and happy or not, but you can. So when you go up for your oral don't care a cent, look the examiner bashfully in the face and smile your best smile and laugh at him. Don't be serious for anything, it won't pay. Students go in with long serious faces which give the examiner dyspepsia and he plucks them. I always went in for making things pleasant for them and induce them to smile or laugh, which made them feel happy and of course overlook mistakes. Try it and you will find the oral a pleasure rather than a bore.

You remember the picture of the ice palace you gave me, well I have it over the mantel-piece. It is much admired by all who see it. The needle case if full of needles, some of which I have had to use.

I had a fractured clavicle to set last week and some wounds to stitch up.

I think I shall have to persuade one of my sisters to come out here; it would be so pleasant for me.

Just this minute a gentleman came in and presented me with a valuable clinical thermometer in a gold case. It was sent me by the manager of the National Bank, Horsham. I attended his little boy when he died of convulsions, cerebral. I scarcely left him for 20 hours, had two other Drs. in who could do no more than I was doing. I feel very much pleased to rec. such a token of regard. Do you know a little thing like that touches my heart in a part that is tender.

I have just a few minutes before mail closes, which if I miss, you will not rec. this letter for two months or more.

In my next letter I shall be able to say what my prospects are to work up a good practice. I have a few good cases on hand, which if they turn out well will give me plenty to do.

I am only on trial, as it were. People look and wonder whether to trust me or not. Once a name is made everything goes smoothly.

Kindly remember me to Mrs. Savage and your people at home.

Wishing you the success that has always attended your efforts, during the coming exams,

I remain yours Sincerely ———————————— — just the same as a year ago.

William C. Little
Warracknabeal

P.S. 1 — I have not time to correct mistakes so be good enough to overlook them.

Wm. C. L.

P.S. 2 — This is the way local papers write up the Drs. in this country. It makes life fun too.

WILLIAM C. LITTLE, M.D., Ch.M.

Member of the College of Physicians and Surgeons, Ontario.

Licentiate Royal College of Surgeons, Edinburgh; and

Fellow of the Obstetrical Society, Edinburgh.

SURGERY:

PHILLIPS - STREET, WARRACKNABEAL

"Terrible ad, isn't it? New Drs. always put in their qualifications. It is not done for show"

(Rec. May 17, 1890)

Warracknabeal
April 10, 1890

My dear Grace,

I received your very welcome letter of Feb. 23 to hand yesterday morning. I also rec. the letter before this one. I began a letter to you about a month ago when lo and behold I found I was too late for the mail. Very often we do not receive notice of the mails until the day before the boat sails. However at that time I was so much taken up with getting furniture, pots, pans and all the other nonsense required to cook a man a meal that my letter would scarcely have been worth reading.

I received the "Globe" all right and the dear handkerchief just as nice and clean as the day you enclosed it. It's a wonder some of the ship mail men did not notice it was in the paper. I knew there was something in it the minute I touched it. It was really kind of you to send it to me and I thank you very much indeed.

Great United States! (a new cuss word) what a correct picture of the Royal and really, after all, the whole description is not overdrawn. I am going to send it to a fellow graduate who came out here 3 yrs. ago.

When I last wrote you I had just received a present of a gold cased thermometer. My name is nicely engraved on it. I am quite proud of it. It is worth six guineas, $30, pretty valuable thing to stick in people's mouths. I only use it on 1st class patients that use a tooth brush at least every morning.

I have had some experience in Australian horse racing during the past two months. My luck has not left me yet for I went into three sweeps and won two and won every bet I made, which were only two. Don't think I am becoming a gambler. Oh no, I am not foolish enough for that — but still it is nice just to bet a £1. for the fun of the thing and it is real fun if you win it.

Well, Grace, I am getting along first class. Some days I have all I can do, not 15 minutes to eat my meals. Last week was my best week in which I made £50 or $250. It would take me two months to make that much in Canada. Yesterday was a busy day, I made $75, of which $50 was cash. I prescribed for 8 patients in the forenoon, drove 22 miles to see a patient in the afternoon. I left at 2 p.m. and got back at 9:30 and visited three patients after that. You could not drive 44 miles in that time in Canada. The country is perfectly level and we never think of allowing a horse to walk.

During my first month I made $200, my 2nd $515 and if this month keeps on, it will be worth $1000. Oh you old Jew, I hear you say, always talking $ and cents. I have had some good cases, which has put me on equal footing with any of the Drs. in this section of the county. My first best hit was a young man with an ulcer on the side of his cheek. He had been treating with 3 other Drs. for over 5 yrs. In despair he was going to Melbourne when some kind friend advised him to see me. The other Drs. diagnosed Epithelioma. I recognized it immediately and told him it was not and that I thought I could cure it. The result was a perfect cure in 21 days. Secret of success, Pot. Iodide in full doses, grn. $\overline{xx}$ t.i.d. This young man was of good family and they were despairing of his life, and he had failed away to a skeleton through brooding over cancer. I told him he could not have a cancer if he tried. I never saw a man gain in flesh so fast. He has a wide connection of friends and they are all singing my praises.

Another interesting case was one of epilepsy in a child 9 yrs. old who had been under a number of Drs. Some days she took 3 and 4 fits. I have been treating her for 8 weeks and she has never had one. If the fits can be stopped for a year she may quite grow out of them.

Drowning people will grasp at straws. I was sent for two weeks ago to see a patient suffering from puerperal fever. She was not expected to live 12 hours. Temp. 103½, pulse 156. They had become dissatisfied with the Dr. in attendance. I wanted to treat the case with him. In my absence some quarrel had taken place as the Dr. had been drinking, so he was dismissed altogether. This all occurred within 3 hrs from [when] I was called first.

I fought with that woman night and day for two days when she suddenly took a change for the better. She had dysentery fearfully bad, which the Dr. did not try to check. The woman was believed to be as good as dead so I gave medicines in no homeopathic doses. Opium grn. $\overline{i}$ repeated every hour until grn. $\overline{iii}$ had been taken to stop dysentery and pain. I tried infusion of Digitalis [oz.] SS combined with [oz.] $\overline{i}$ of Fl. Ext. Ergotae, repeated in 4 hours (not by the mouth) to slow the heart, Quinine grn. $\overline{viii}$ by the mouth and grn. $\overline{vi}$ injected under the skin to reduce temperature. I sponged the body and limbs with the best whiskey every 2 hours. In two hours I saw a change for the better. She will be able to be up in a day or two. This case will be worth $2000 to me this year.

An old Dr. who lives 40 miles away from here helped me a lot. I was called to a case of Uremic convulsions from chronic Bright's disease. I told the friends I could not save her and that I would do all I could for her, and as I was only young in the profession it might be more satisfactory to get the opinion of some other Dr. This was my 2nd consultation. The old Dr. examined her and said I was right in my diagnosis and then asked me for my treatment. He told the friends I had done all that could be done and also added that my head was level, that I had done more for her than he could have done. The woman's brother told me this. You may be sure I felt grateful to the old Dr.

I get a good deal to do in surgery. Yesterday I reduced a dislocated shoulder, Saturday set a fractured tibia, the Wed. before amputated a finger, a few days before stitched up a child's hand that had 3 of the metacarpal bones cut through. They had taken the child to another Dr. the night before. He just stuck some sticking plaster on and left the metacarpal bones sticking out through the wound and the arteries untied. The child was nearly bled to death. I stitched it up beautifully after twisting the arteries. The wound is healing up very fast. I cut a young man's tonsils off abt. a month ago. He had been doctoring for yrs. with sore throat. As soon as I examined him I told him they would have to come off, to which he agreed. I sent away for a Tonsilatome, cut them off and charged him $15 for the job. His throat is cured.

You will require to have yours cut off as they are 3 times too large and you will always be subject to sore throat so long as you have those inflamed and enlarged tonsils. They are no good anyway, so far as I can find out. Probably they are useful in keeping the throat moist.

I have bought a lovely pair of horses. I shall send you a picture of my house, horses and carriage some time. Also a picture of how Australians store grain. I have been successful in getting a splendid housekeeper. I could not get a better in all Australia. I never saw her when I engaged her. I sent her a telegram that I would pay her $250 a year. She is a lady very well educated, can make a good *PIE* and get a good dinner. She is not a bit inquisitive, no gossip and keeps my breakfast warm when I don't get up early. I often sleep to 10 in the morning. I have got such a comfortable bed, the best I could get and I do enjoy it. Some nights I do not get to bed at all. I was called 3 nights after each other, first night I had just undressed, 2nd I had ½ undressed and the 3rd I had ½ my collar unbuttoned; I looked at the cosy bed and said, "Darn them, why don't they get sick in the day time."

I have only attended four confinement cases, all forcep cases. The women here don't send for a Dr. until they find that all efforts of nature are of no avail.

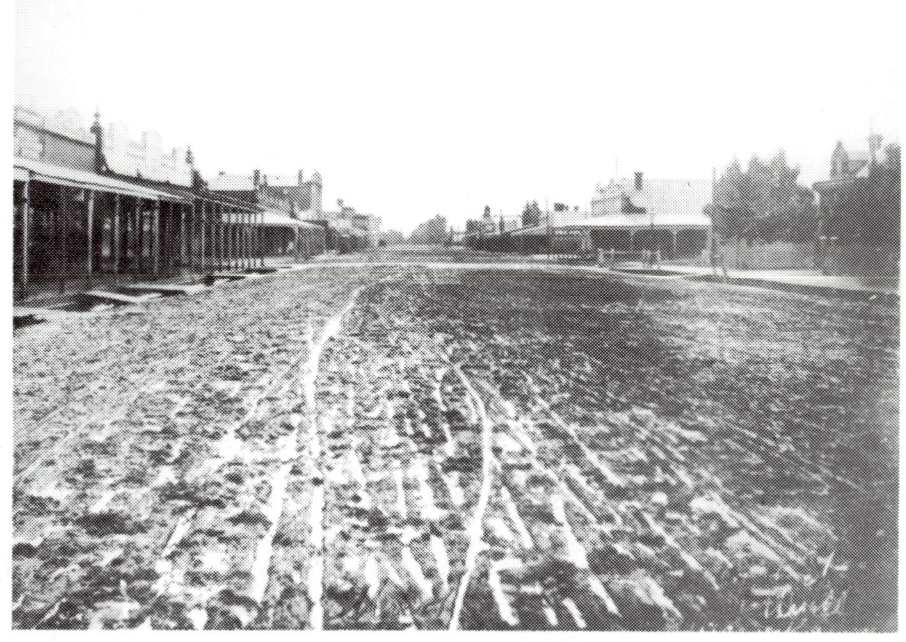

Scott Street, Warracknabeal, in Winter

So you have read "The Silence of Dean Maitland." How funny that we should both have read it about the same time. Did tears come in your eyes or a lump in your throat? It worked on my feelings very much. What a mean way he took to shirk the murder by wearing his friend's coat. I felt very sorry for his sister. I am reading a book "Looking Backward" by Edward Bellamy. A man goes to sleep under mesmeric influence in Boston in the year 1887 and wakes up in yr. 2000. I think you would like it. [25]

I occasionally read a wild sensational story to make my blood curdle and my hair stand on end so that the air may get at the roots and prevent me from becoming bald headed.

Oh, I must not forget to tell you I have got a new name for you which I hope you will like. Supposing I would leave you to guess. Well, that would be as bad as yourself and Miss Demerest when you were calling me "By Gingo" or some such name. Well, your name is a nice name and called after an animal you would just feel like hugging if you saw it: when it is tame it loves to cozy itself on your knee and have its soft coat gently stroked and you never know one minute what it will do the next. This very affectionate animal is known by the name of *"Possum."* Now, how do you like your new name? You do look like a possum when you have your circular on with the fur side out. I quite admire your choice of a friend in Miss Henderson. I liked her very much indeed.

Shuttleworth gave quite a nice little address at the banquet. Have you met him yet? He is so bashful.

You say you have been very demure this winter, well take my advice, don't be demure any longer, you will only spoil your looks and make yourself unhappy. I tell you Grace, if you practise medicine you will find then that it is quite early enough to begin to think about being serious. When you are called to a case and you find you are as weak as a child to save a life then you feel what seriousness really means. I was called to attend a man with pneumonia of both lungs. When I examined him I knew I was perfectly helpless to save him as it had gone too far before I was called. The mother is dead and the three daughters pled with me to save their father. I saw him three times and he died while I was there the 3rd time. I could do nothing to improve his condition. I suppose I shall get accustomed to such things but I could not sleep.

The weather is perfectly serene now and I am quite myself again. I have gained in weight and feel fit for anything. When I get too much surplus energy I go and have a game of billiards; you should see me bang the balls about and sometimes I send them whizzing off the table. I don't know how to play but for all I am very lucky at pocketing the balls. I bang ahead and the balls roll into the pockets, much to my amusement and of those looking on. They call me the lucky shot, that I always win by flukes. I resent that and assert that I play a scientific American game.

I only play when I am feeling full of old Nick and I suppose that's how I get along so well.

This is the most egotistical letter I ever saw penned. Don't you think it is full of 👁 👁 . I do a great deal of reading. I am getting Pepper's System of Medicine, and Safons on the nose and throat.

I am sorry you did not get the clinic I sent from Edinburgh. It might be sticking around the post office in Montreal. I am taking Byron Bromwell's clinics. I much prefer them to the journals. I prefer the sound advice of a thoroughly clever Dr. to the vague theories of a dozen experimentalists.

I must go to bed and finish this tomorrow.

Glad to hear you rec. so many birthday gifts. So you got a gold thermometer too.

It will just be about a year since I saw you last by the time you rec. this letter. I wish I could join you in your holidays at the sea side, but such cannot be at present. Something tells me that we shall meet again but when, where and how shall be decided by the wheels of time and fate.

One part of my life I have quite decided on and that is to take holidays every year and every 5th year to take six months' holidays to travel and learn as much about the world as possible. Nothing like enjoying life as you go along. I fancy you think me a happy go lucky fellow who never views life from the dark and serious side. So serious a view do I take of life that I firmly believe if we do not use all our mortal powers to find the bright and sunny side of life, we will be sure to find the dark side and when we come to wind up our affairs, we will feel we have defeated the very object for which we were created. My darkest hours are very often my brightest hours, for I well know when the sunshine does come, and come it must, I enjoy it all the more.

No more moralizing for I really believe I am getting La Grippe. I have a pain in my head, my back aches, cold chills are running down my spinal column. These symptoms have all come on during the past hour. I wonder where the bright side of La Grippe is. I fancy it is when someone else has it and they pay me to attend them and the 2nd theory is the sooner I get it the sooner I shall be over it.

La Grippe is raging in Melbourne and is fast travelling in this direction. If I get any worse I shall take grn. $\overline{viii}$ of quinine, [oz.] $\overline{iv}$ of whiskey and Dover's Pow. [26] and go to bed. You should have told me what was considered the best treatment for it in Canada. A number of Melbourne cases have developed Pneumonia and some have proved fatal.

You will, I have no doubt, learn a great deal with the Dr. you mention. That means of course you are not going to accept my offer. Let me know the results of Exams. You will pass flying, no trouble in the world about it.

I must close as my head is getting worse. I can scarcely see. Give my best remembrances to your mother and sisters, also to your little nephew if he can understand.

I hope you will have a pleasant holiday and no mosquitoes to bite you. Pyrethrum is the stuff to paralyse them.

Now goodbye and be good, as a friend of mine used to say to me, and remember I like you as well as I did a year ago. Don't think me foolish for telling you that, for did I feel otherwise I would tell you also.

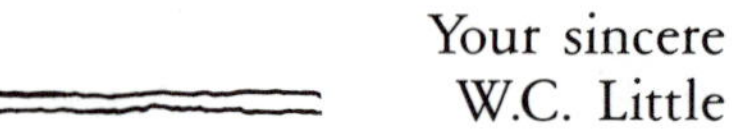

Your sincere
W.C. Little

P.S. Evening. My temp. is 101 and I have a fearful pain in back and head. I have taken Quinine, Dover's, coffee and whiskey and am going to bed. If I get worse I shall send for a Dr. I shall give this to the housekeeper to post. Sick and all as I feel, I have prescribed for 12 patients today. If I don't shake off this mortal coil, I shall tell you what is the matter with me in my next — and if I do, I shall bequeath you my engraved gold cased thermometer. Don't you think me generous, ha! ha! I must go to bed. Good-bye.

(Rec. July 13, 1890)
Ans. (?)

Warracknabeal
June 8, 1890

My dear Grace,

It really seems as if it were six months since I wrote you last. I really hope you won't think me a negligent sinner for not writing last mail. I missed it through the papers not publishing the time the vessel sailed early enough. I was going to write you by England but this letter in any case will reach you first.

When I wrote you last the spasms of La Grippe were coming on, and on they did come in proper style. I was as sick as a horse, temp. 102½, headache, backache and a fearful cough. Strange to say, I was the first to get it. I believe you sent it to me in your letter, no one else had it in the town for three weeks after I had it. I did not make my will. How fortunate I was to have it first. I got quite well to look after the others. I had the groom sponge my back with Camphor and whiskey every morning until pains all left.

Oh, I have been so busy that I scarcely get time to sleep. Just fancy, I made $1500 last month, and something like $800 the month before. I shall make $1200 this month. I wish you had accepted my offer and come and helped me. I have frequently examined 20 patients in one day. Wouldn't I have been a fool to have remained in Canada. I make more in one month than lots of Drs. do in Canada in one year. I charged $75 the other night for one visit and the man thanked me and said he expected to have to pay more. I can remember how astounded I was when I heard of Dr. Sullivan charging $40–60 for going 50 miles to see a patient. Oh, how I longed to be able to do that. So far my practice has been of the most satisfactory kind. I have been quite flattered several times by patients coming 70 and 80 miles on the train to see me.

I bought another pair of horses the other day as one pair could not stand the work. Well, I must stop talking about myself, it is vain. I fancy beginning practice is something like newly married life, wonderfully interesting and exciting. Well, I shall settle down to real sober practice after awhile and will not get excited.

I was so delighted last mail to see a paper from home with your name marked all around and "Clever Girl" written beneath it, stating you won

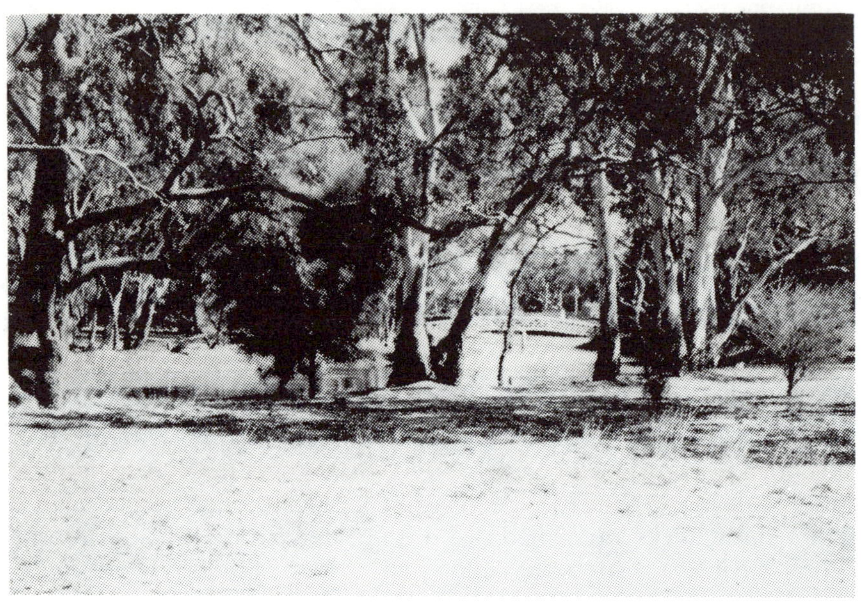

*"I have often wished you could drop down here just to see what heavenly weather
Australia can boast of sometimes and to have one of our long, long talks"*

the scholarship. My sister sent the paper. Well, I am quite pleased with you.
I knew you would win if you tried. I would have bet $50 to 1 on you. I
was pleased to see Miss Henderson also came to the front. You see I took
in your mental calibre about right when I said Porpoise and Hen were the
cleverest girls in the W.M.C.K.

I am sure you would be glad to get home from K[ingston]. It is such
a pokey place. Did you go to Lachute this year? You will be having lovely
weather now, everything beautiful and the climate all that could be desired.

I have quite changed my feelings abt. Australia. The climate is a
perfect heaven. I often go for a 2 or 3 mile drive first thing in the morning.
How I do enjoy it. The atmosphere, the air, the sun, the trees and birds
all combined make me feel truly happy. All this I enjoy in silence and alone.
I have often wished you could drop down here just to see what heavenly
weather Australia can boast of sometimes and to have one of our long, long
talks.

At present I have not made any friends. By friends I mean persons I can confide in. No, no, I am all business. To be a successful Dr. a very peculiar combination is required — Patients must be kept in their place. No matter how well I am acquainted with a person when he comes to the surgery, I make him feel he does not know me. I forget that I know him. Examine, talk and act as if he were a perfect stranger. I could do it with my own brother and I can tell you I am very very thankful that I have such a gift. Patients must never be allowed to become familiar. Write that motto in large letters in your surgery and read it every day. So soon as a patient becomes familiar he will lose faith in you. Keep patients like servants, in their place, and they will respect you. I gave a man a good send [up] the other evening when a party of us were sitting in a public parlor having a social time. He related a great number of symptoms he complained of and wound up by wanting to know what I would do in such a case. I said I would most certainly consult a Dr. I immediately turned the topic of conversation and left the man to study out what I meant. Never prescribe for patients under such circumstances. If you do, you lower yourself.

I had rather an enjoyable day last Tuesday. The Governor, Lord Hopetoun,[27] was here. I was at the banquet, etc.

I shall send you a photo of his Excellency as he landed after two days' hard riding, his clothes and face all spattered with mud. I shall also send you a photo of my surgery and myself standing around somewhere.

I think you promised me a cabinet photo the next time you got any taken. I shall be delighted to receive it.

Oh, my cousin Dr. Cross has gone home. He was going to call on you. I hope you were at home for I am sure he would tell you some funny yarns. You might not like him at first, but on longer acquaintance you would find him a superior fellow. He is coming out here in August or September. I shall try and meet him in Melbourne on his arrival.

Oh, I am doing a pretty good eye practice here. I picked up a great deal from Connell besides what I learned in Edinburgh. I have cured a case that was under the best eye Dr. in Melbourne. She was sent home worse than when she went away. I cured her in 3 weeks. Whenever you undertake an eye case look to the general health first, and if anything is wrong treat that first. In treating granulated lids I clip off the granulations with a fine pair of shears. I then apply to the *outside* of the lid silver nitrate pencil, which acts as a counter irritant. It produces rather an amusing effect, for the lid is blackened. I use Lapis Divinus[28] for the granulations.

The F.O.S. [29] is bringing me in a good deal of gynecological work. I had *two cases* of post partum hemorrhage in one week. 1st case, the child was born a few min. before I got there, the woman nearly dead. 2nd case, primipara delivered with forceps. I had an awful job to get it stopped. I never knew I could be frightened with blood before. I never want such an experience again. If you ever have a case, put your hand into the uterus and bear down, compressing the abdominal aorta. at the same time instructing the nurse to give two drachms of ergot. The blood would not stop, because the uterus would not contract. I thought of the abdominal aorta and pressed firmly on it and with gratifying results. This was the first time I ever felt myself weaken or tremble. I could not help it and could not understand why I couldn't. I felt strange for 2 hrs. after.

June 9th, just one hour until train leaves to catch the boat. I feel quite upset this morning. I have for the last 3 or 4 days been attending a Dr.'s wife here when yesterday I discovered the cause of her illness. Morphia habit. The Dr. is also addicted to it. I am going to do my best to cure them of it. The Dr.'s wife is like a Maniac this morning for want of it. When I told her I discovered what her trouble was, she positively denied it. I bared her arms and also thighs and showed her the punctures of the needle. At last she admitted it. Hell is nothing compared with such a curse.

I have all the practice to myself now so that I will now be very busy. There are patients in the waiting room but I must finish this letter.

Have you really decided to leave the W.M.C.K.? Whatever you do don't take Trinity College Toronto degree. [30] It is no good outside of Ontario or Canada. Trinity is looked upon in this country as a bogus college. It seems they have been showering down degrees of all kinds for a consideration.

Well, if you finish in Kingston and come out first I'll promise you something you will like. However you know what is best for yourself.

If ever you expect to make $50,000 a year, you will have to come to Australia and I think Melbourne will be the best place. You can easily make $5000 a year in Melbourne as Lady Drs. are rather a novel thing out here. [31] The fees are so much better than at home. I see papers from Kingston with recent Grad. names. Jack Shannon did very well. I fancy Jack will make quite a Ladies Dr. and of course must necessarily do well.

There are lots of Drs. out here who cannot make a living simply because they have not means to begin on and have not a taking manner. Do you know Grace, my life seems to have undergone a change since I came here. A week does not seem a day to me, it is work, work all the time. The Australians call it Grafting — a new word for you.

You are the only person in Canada that I have let know how well I am doing. It would be better for you not to say anything about it to others, as it might be the means of bringing other Drs. out here and when they would come they might find themselves very much disappointed, for there are lots of Drs. out here who cannot find a place to practise and are simply travelling around the country with Insurance agents, making what they can.

Now goodbye and be good and don't work too hard. I wish I could spend a holiday with you this summer, we would have a jolly time.

Your sincere
W.C. Little

(Rec. Aug 9, 1890
Ans. (?) — Les Eboulements)

Warracknabeal
July 6, 1890

My dear Possum,

Your combined letter of May 6 & 18 came to hand one week ago. It was on Saturday night — after doing a *very* hard day's work. I felt so tired that I lay back in a huge rocking chair I have, just to dream a little over the past and so on, when the groom rapped at the door and called out, "Foreign letters, sir." I jumped to my feet and forgot about dreams and weariness so eager was I to know the contents of them. I read yours first and I do not know when a letter made me feel so happy. It was so honest and girl-like that I for the time felt myself as if in your company. There are letters and letters, but none so dear so refreshing to read as those which give a perfect picture of the writer's feelings whether joyous or otherwise.

I think it is Victor Hugo who says, "It is a treat reserved only for angels to be privileged to look into a maiden's room." Granting that he is correct, how flattered I should feel, and so I do. I laughed so at the drawing of your room. It is very funny when you think of it. Why I can just imagine you up there reading, thinking, "jabbering" as you call it, and all kinds of performances such as you used to go through at Allens. The worst of it is when I think of you I think of the room and fancy you in it — in fact if I had not thought of it, I would never have you out of it.

So my cousin called on you and I am sure you thought him a peculiar fellow. He is an odd card until you know him. He will say anything, whatever comes in his head. You say, "Cheeky," well, yes he is, but he means no harm. I remember one night at a party, things were a bit dull, because the good people of the house were very religious and thought the singing of hymns and so on were proper amusements. I felt bored and so did Cross. All at once Cross jumped up and said, "Let us go. Let us get out of this hole." What a look passed around the room. He felt it very much afterwards. He would be very sure to concoct any amount of nonsense to tell you. Hasn't he an odd laugh? I do so like to hear him laugh.

To speak my mind, rain, mud and devils seem to be the state of the elements tonight. Every step I hear I fancy it is coming for me hence the word with the "d" in. I do hope I have not to go out tonight, as it is fearfully dark and the rain is pouring down. I am so comfortable where I am — a beautiful fire on, a nice cushioned chair and your good company present in the spirit — so I do not want to be disturbed.

What a trip I had the night before last. I was called to see a patient — 22 miles and alas when I got there she and the child were dead. "Post-partum" from "Placenta Marginata." I felt so sad to think had I been there I could have saved her life. I rode on horseback, left at 5 p.m. and got back at 3 a.m. — 44 miles. I am so sore I do not [know] what position to take to get comfort. I am all sore. It is only lately I have taken to horseback riding. I am getting to be a good rider. I love to go fast. I did 10 miles in 1 hr. and 5 minutes the other day. Patient died also.

Now for my grievances — I am wild about the state of things obstetrically in this country. Women undertake to confine (other women) who are so d— ignorant they don't know enough to wash their face, much less their hands. They happen to have attended a few cases where the patient could have got on quite well alone and then they advertise themselves as being very clever and even canvass for the job. I have had no less than 8 cases the result of such ignorant ignorance, three of whom died — two cases Cellulitis, one sub-involution and Cellulitis and three that died Post-partum and Puerperal fevers, the others mild septicemia.

The manager of the paper interviewed me the other day as to the cause of septic fever. After a brief explanation I said that there is only one woman in Australia capable of confining women and that was a lady Dr. in Melbourne. He said did I mean to say trained nurses were incompetent and I said I will put it a little stronger, that no woman other than a Dr., no trained nurse no matter what amount of hospital experience she has had, is capable of conducting a confinement, that she in serious complications is as helpless as the unborn child. [32] I further said that any woman under-taking such cases, excepting where a Dr. could not be got, was guilty of malpractice and further, any woman who if she learns the information I have given you undertakes such cases and the patient dies, she is guilty of the highest crime. The reporter thanked me for the information, & said I had made him a wiser man & that he expected an increase in his family before long and would like me to attend. He told me he had foolishly listened to old women's self praise.

To give you an idea of what ignorance I meet with, a man consulted me for a cough his wife had after confinement. I prescribed, but said I am afraid she has something worse the matter. I told him, if she were at all feverish or chilly a Dr. had better see her. I was asked two days afterwards to see her. I had 10 miles to go. When I got there I met a big self praised midwife who informed me that the patient was quite well, that she had her sitting in the rocking chair, that it was the husband that was anxious. "Well," I said, "I must see the patient after coming 10 miles." "Oh yes, by all means." I examined her, found her temp. 104½, pulse 140. She was quite delirious, talking very jolly, which the nurse took for health. They wanted to know what I thought when I was about to leave. "Well," I said, "I suppose you want to know the truth?" They all said "yes." "Well," I said, "she won't live more than 4 or 5 days." She died the 5th day.

I mentioned in my last letter about the Dr.'s wife being a confirmed opium taker. Well, she died of Bright's disease. Her husband attended her to within one week of her death and yet did not detect the kidney disease nor yet did he know she took morphia. I of course kept the morphia habit quiet or the public would think she killed herself. She was fond of drink. She was only 27 yrs. old, good looking and accomplished.

The lesson to be learned from the above is never to undertake to treat yourself or your intimate friends, particularly your own family, for you will be very likely to treat lightly serious diseases and exaggerate milder ailments, just as liable to do it that way as the right way. All Drs. who undertake to treat their own families make such mistakes.

I am still doing well. Practice is not all like the last pages. There are bright pages; patients [who] are very sick or think so, get well, they are thankful to the Dr. for the good care he gave them. They in the fullness of their hearts send other patients and so life goes on with a few little dark spots to mar but a 1000 times more sunshine, which helps to obliterate the darkness.

I get a great deal of credit for a prognosis I gave. I was called to see an old woman with mitral regurgitation. I told the husband, sons and daughters that I could do very little for her, that she would improve under treatment for a time. I told the daughters to be kind to her, that they would not have her long. I then told them the course the disease would take and what to do. She lived 8 weeks and died as I had told them. The people in that part think I know everything.

I made $175 in one day, $40 in the surgery, the rest by long drives — two confinement cases where the nurses failed; one, the child was rather large, forceps, the other the midwife could not remove the placenta. Both cases did well.

I am doing a good eye practice. Last month eye practice was worth $200. I did an operation last Monday for Trichiasis and Entropion.[33] I removed an elliptical piece of skin from the upper lid, excised the underside of the lid at the junction of conjunction with skin and stitched it up. It is going to effect a cure. I expect a patient in next week to have his cross eyes straightened. I have several Pterygiums[34] to remove. Do you remember when I had that small one removed off my eye? The above operation I charge $50 for. I did an operation today — cut out an indolent ulcer.

I have no less than 7 or 8 cases of phthisis, all of which are improving. I paint the chest with iodine, give a comb. of Glycerine, Brandy and Menthol, also Ol. Murrhual, Spts. Turpentine, chloroform and menthol combined.

> Rx Ol Terebinthinae ʒij
> Menthol gra IV
> Chloroforme ʒj
> Ol Murrhua aʒ ʒviij
> Sig ʒj mercuril ls ʒij ℈d.
> after meals

The above is one of my own concoctions and I like it very much. Last month's practice was worth something over $1000, which is not bad for a "new chum."

I am sincerely sorry to learn that Miss Bennett is so poorly. Poor girl, I hope she will come through the operation all right. I quite agree with you that she is a very fine girl, but still there was something between us besides the mesmerism, which if it had been removed would have made us very good friends I think.

I often wonder what happened to Mrs. Walker. I am sure there is something or other. She has a grudge against me for something, probably because I used to take your part. Anyway, she never answered any letters I ever sent her. I wrote her from Montreal last. Dr. Demerest — how funny! I fancy I hear her tell her patients in her droll way, "Open your mouth, stick out your tongue, you have got liver complaint."

If I could say anything nice for you to tell Miss Bennett, I would do so, but then I don't know what to say. The right word in the right place is so cheering, but then if you get it in the wrong place, how disagreeable. Let me see. Tell her I am so sorry she is ill, and that if I could possibly in any way make her suffering less, I would gladly do it. Tell her to be brave as women can be brave and she will come through the operation all right and that I shall be pleased to hear of her speedy recovery.

I am glad you like your new name. Well, the untamed possum is a mischievious little animal. It will run up a tree, sit on a limb and laugh at you as much to say, "Catch me if you can."

So you still think that I think you won't make much of a Dr. ha! ha! Please read that part of my letter again and if you can't see the nicest piece of praise in it you ever got, I'll quit. If I say you will be admired more as a lady than a Dr. and then further back or further ahead or somewhere, yes even in your palmacological chart, positively assert that many will sit at your feet to learn the healing art (which latter part will come true next winter if you choose), is evidence of no ordinary medical ability. Now ain't you sorry I have to explain it to you?

My first housekeeper had to go home on acct. of illness. She was a good woman and a lady, but in many senses did not suit me exactly. I could not treat her as a servant. She dined with me, which I did not like always. Besides, we must talk and she would hear everything; besides she sometimes felt her position, that it was hard to be cook and housekeeper combined without losing caste. Well, she had to go home and I have a good housekeeper now who dines in the kitchen and I dine alone. She suits me well so I shall keep her. She is abt. 40–45, Scotch and a Presbyterian & always addresses me as Dr. or Sir, always has everything in apple pie order for me. If I am out late she leaves a good fire on and supper on the table & calls me — "Dr., it is nine o'clock," which time I generally get up. Her name is Miss Matheson. I call her Flora, which I think she likes. Well now, what do you think of her?

I have a few gentlemen friends you might like to know about. Mr. Grantly, Editor of Warrack. Herald, very jolly company and has a nice wife. I go to his home and smoke a cigar and get the latest news. 2nd, Mr. Oakley, a young lawyer, very fine fellow, lively, lots of common sense, likes a good time but does not go to extremes. I play him billiards frequently. Mr. Phillips, the leading man of the town, has the finest house in the town & a pretty wife, has a billiard table in the house, which I frequently play on.[35] She has helped me a great deal. I prescribed for his wife about a week ago and she got better. Mr. Booth, English Church — a young man, likes a game of billiards, smokes cigars and pipe, calls on me occasionally to have a smoke, and a cup of coffee. We often chew the rag until 12 p.m. and 1 a.m.

Then there is old mother Nuskie who says I am the wonder of the age. She thinks she is dying from snake bites which she never got 22 yrs. ago. I tell her if ever she feels like biting herself or anyone else, to come

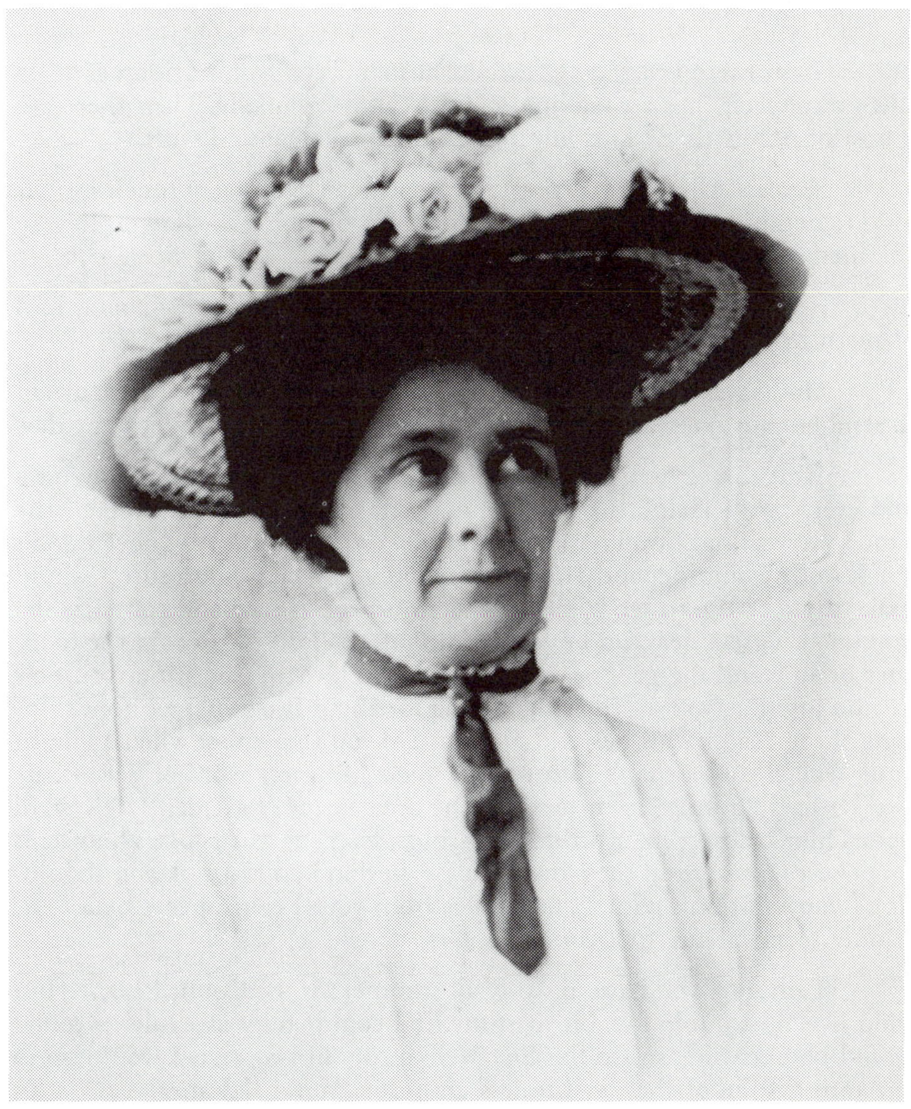

"If I am out late she leaves a good fire on and supper on the table. . . . Her name is Miss Matheson. I call her Flora, which I think she likes"

to me and I will give her medicine to stop her. I ask her if she is quite sure she did not swallow a snake.

Then there is another old woman that calls me Dr. 20 times in a minute, who imagines her children are all dying from nothing and eternally wants them to take medicine.

Then there is a Mrs. O. whose husband is a commission agent — sings very nicely, has a cozy home and I call occasionally. Then there are a host of others that I am only professionally acquainted with.

So Miss Abbott[36] has not forgotten me. Thanks very much for her kind remembrance. Tell her I congratulate her on being so clever as to take the medal. Miss Howard I also remember as being a good *horseman*.

How is your little nephew getting along? I suppose he has a mouthful of teeth by this time and will soon be able to talk to you.

Mrs. Savage I hope is enjoying good health. You know I am afraid to send her any nice messages. Mr. Savage might be in Australia some day.

Well, Grace, we have had quite a long talk tonight about anything and everything. Thank the Lord there wasn't a soul to disturb me all the time I was writing. I wonder if we would feel strange if we met now. I don't think so. It would depend altogether when and where. I am sure I would make some excuse to see your room. I am sure it is nice and comfortable. You know a great deal can be learned about a person just seeing the room they occupy and the general arrangement. Well, I think if I met you now I could interest [you in] chewing the rag for about two weeks without stopping. I can read hands better than ever. Do you remember when I taught you? Well, I told a man's fortune last week and every word of it was true and he lives 70 miles from here. He believes in me. I accidently knew all about him before, which I didn't in your case. The great joke about it is he believes in me, and the worst of it is you don't and I think you should, don't you? To think I am 12,000 miles from you. I can scarcely believe it. It only seems about 100 to me.

I am sorry you have to study all summer for the Council exams, but then it is no trouble for you to study. If I could study as easily as you, I would be practising in Collins St., Melbourne; in two years I would go to the top in spite of the devil unless ambition would slay me.

Now Grace, don't work so hard. You have done enough to entitle you to three months' holidays. A healthy body, rosy cheeks, good spirits, lots of fun and apple pie are worth far more to you than an over-worked brain. Glad to hear you are still keeping *fat*.

So goodbye. Yours as always,
W.C. Little

P.S. 1 — I am going to write Cross this mail. I shall tell him you think him very jolly.
P.S. 2 — When I went to fold the letter I found this sheet a blank. It is bed time, being 12:10.

Oh, the photos I promised you have not been taken yet. I shall mail you some of the town views, how grain is stacked, and will send the others later. Oh, a man called today and wants his 12-yr. old daughter to have her picture taken on my verandah with me standing near her. I have cured her of Epilepsy for the time at least. She consulted me Feb. 14 and has only had 2 since. She had been having 3 & 4 a day.

What a funny idea.

This is Sunday, but I did not go to church.

Monday Morning, July 7th

Dear Possum,

I got a good night's sleep and feel very much better — not quite so sore this morning. Thinking you never saw a Gum tree or Eucalyptus tree, I enclose two or three leaves for you to smell and chew if you like. One of them you may give to your sister Mrs. Savage. I think they have a lovely smell, probably the smell & taste will be all gone before they reach you.

It is just an hour till the mail goes out so I shall have to hurry and get the photos I promised you. If you don't get them, it is because I could not get them in time.

I hope you will get along nicely with Dr. Smith or "Happy" as you call him. If he were not married, I would be feeling a little jealous of him.

I won't have the time to read over this letter and make corrections, so will just ask you to do it for me.

A patient just came in to say he would come on Wednesday to have two Pterygii removed, $75 for the job. If I get enough to do, I shall be rich someday. I don't care much for money, still it's very useful in its way. If I were rich, I would ask you to take a trip around the world with me. Of course we would have to have Mrs. Savage along too, ha! ha!

Good bye and *be good.*   W.C.L.

P.S. Possums live on Gum leaves, so you will have to eat your leaf. I enclose a little one for Miss Abbott.

Letters with pepper fronds, gum leaves and "the little bamboon"

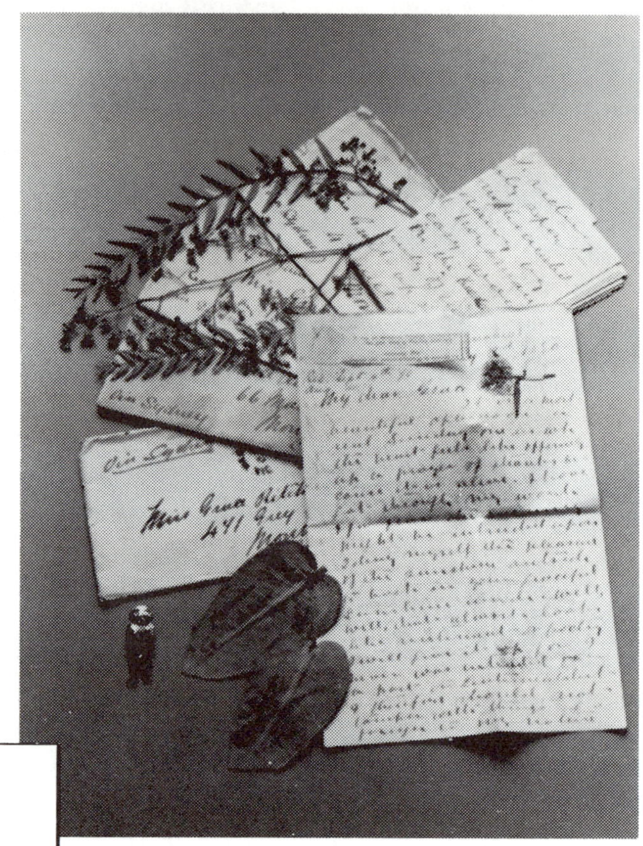

"While at the buddhist temple I bought two little Gods, offerings to his Godship Buddha, one of which I enclose to you. It is pure silver. You can keep the little baboon in your pocketbook to keep ghosts away or anything else you like. I think it would be better if it were dressed up a little, but I shall leave that for your dainty fingers to do"

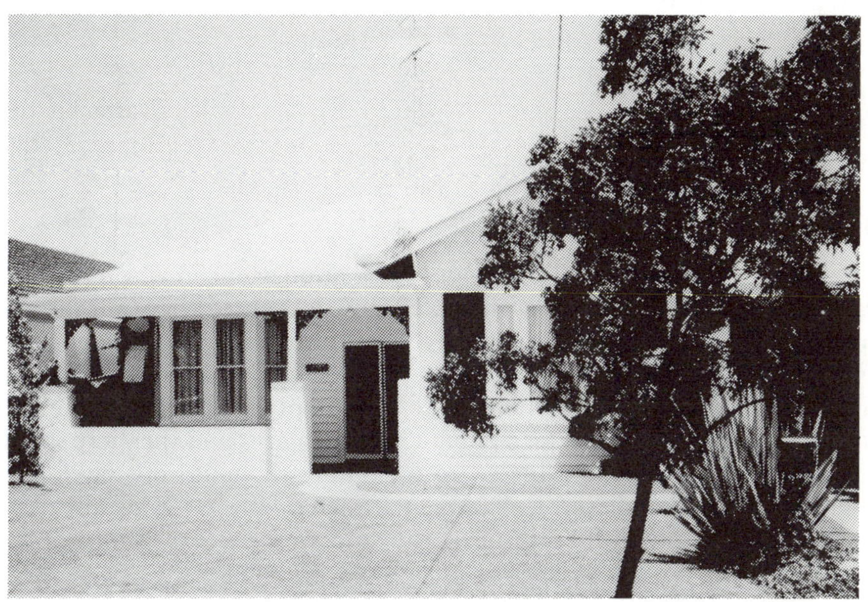

Dr. Little's house as it appears today

Dear Grace,

I got the photos. No 1 is a bullock team, the way farmers bring their grain to market. No. 2, Then the grain is stacked at the station. $\frac{1}{11}$ of all the wheat grown in Victoria was put down at Warracknabeal station. No. 3 is a perspective of $\frac{1}{2}$ of the town. The house with the mark $\triangle$ on the roof is my surgery, etc. The little square house at the back is the kitchen and housekeeper's room. The front of my house has a nice garden with vines and pepper trees. The three views unnumbered are views of the river. I shall some time send you a photo of myself, house, horses and carriage.

Let me know how you like them.

No more at present.

Yours sincerely,
W.C.L.

P.S. Did you get the Australasian paper I sent you in January with the native Maiden's picture?

(Rec. Sept. 4, 1890)
Ans. do (?)

Warracknabeal
August 3, 1890

My Dear Grace,

It is a most beautiful afternoon, a real Sunday one in which the heart feels like offering up a prayer of thanks because it is alive. I have got through my work and for fear the evening might be intruded upon, I deny myself the pleasure of the sunshine outside to bask in your graceful sunshine inside. Well, well, that almost looks like sentiment or poetry. I will give it up for I never was intended for a poet or sentimentalist and therefore should not tamper with things so foreign to my nature. I should not say foreign to my nature, for I believe I feel and am attracted by what is beautiful and sentimental but my dull brain never can find words to express it as many others can.

Your last letter of June 17th came to hand abt. 5 days ago. You appear to be happy, but where in mischief did you get anaemia? Well, if you don't know, I do. Do you remember me telling you, you had a bad throat and I think I mentioned in one of my letters you should have your throat operated on? Well, your throat is the cause either directly or ind. of the trouble. The oxidation of the blood is interfered with, so how could you help losing color. Your tonsils are very much hypertrophied, which extends to the Eustachian tubes and interferes with your hearing.

So Miss Abbott sent me her love with a pinch of salt — was she afraid it would spoil on the way that she added the salt? Just fancy love or a kiss carefully salted down, packed in a box and shipped to Australia free of duty. Now don't you tell her this — it was only the way it occurred to me.

Well, you have a wonderfully intelligent kitten — what do you call it? Mark Antoni after Lilian's in the "Silence of Dean Maitland"? Do you know I often think of Lilian. I shall never forget her beautiful character and particularly her wonderful powers over animals. Do you think you could tame wild cats, bad horses and last if not least, fractious youth?

I have just finished reading a most beautiful novel, "Infelice," written by Augusta Wilson. I know you will like it. Your little heart will go pitta pat when Madame Orme appears before a Paris audience in Kenilworth — it is simply grand. Her daughter Regina you will like and were I asked to portray a man after your own heart, a man I know your very nature could not help but be drawn to, "Mr. Palmer," the lawyer. If you have not read "Infelice" let me know how you like it when you do. Oh, how I would like to join you in your holiday in the French village, where I could just run wild for a few days. How I feel like kicking over the traces, throwing off the harness and just have a free and happy time. I have to be so precise, always look and act the Dr., give the most solemn advice with a long serious face, sympathize and show feeling for poor mortals' troubles, when in my inmost soul I could laugh at them. The very old devil takes possession of me sometimes. There is a Dr. here who is forever complaining. He brings his troubles to me, has me feel his pulse, examine his throat, etc. He came to me about a week ago just shortly after [I had received] a summons to appear in *court* for riding on the footpath. I was out of temper and as the Dr. is an awful bore, he did not put me in any better humor. He stuck out his arm for me to feel his pulse, at the same time saying, "Oh Dr. I believe I am going to die." "Die," I said, "why don't you, it would do you good. Lie down on the sofa and let me see you try to die. I'll bet you five guineas you couldn't die if you tried." Those two sentences relieved me of my temper. I sat down and had a good laugh at him and he joined me. He has not troubled me since, for I think he understood me quite well, that I considered he was shamming.

I did ride on the footpath, but I didn't appear in court. I employed an Irish lawyer to paralyse the informant, to call him all the names he could think of, to simply roar at him, after which to plead guilty for me. The whole town is in raptures over the defense. The informant, I am told, stood with his mouth open, his hair on end and afterwards left the court room not knowing which end of him was uppermost. You see I had two amusements out of one disagreeability.

I may as well tell you some more of my troubles. In my last, I told you what kind of nurses I had to put up with. A sample — I was called to a case of convulsions in a married woman, which occurred shortly after weaning the child. I could not at first make out the cause. It was either epilepsy or uremia.

I came home leaving word for the husband to bring me some of the urine as soon as possible, which he did in the course of a few hrs. She was suffering from Bright's Disease. I gave philocarpen, etc. and instructed the nurses to keep her warm by putting hot water bottles or warm bricks to her feet. When I called to see the patient next morning, I smelt cloth burning. I immediately pulled down the bed clothes, which I found on fire. The bricks were so hot they set fire to the cloths that were put around them. One leg

[Wannehanaheu?]

Aug 2d 1870

Rec. Sept 4th '70
Ans. [done?]

My dear Grace

It is a most beautiful afternoon — a real Sunday one in which the heart feels like offering up a prayer of thanks because it is alive. I have sat through my work & for fear this Evening might be intruded upon I deny myself the pleasure of the sunshine outside to bask in your graceful [sunshine?] inside. Well, well, but almost looks like sentiment — or poetry I will give it up for I never was intended to — a poet or sentimentalist & therefore should not tamper with things & foreign to my nature of patient between knee and ankle was roasted to the bone. Where the hot water bottles were put the flesh was cooked. All the blankets were burned through. I told them to hold the hot water bottles to their face before putting them to the patient and to hold the bricks in their hands to be sure they would not be too hot. The above were the results. The patient died while I was there. She was quite unconscious and therefore did not feel the burning. The two women who were attending her replaced the blankets and none but themselves and you and I know of it. What do you think of such a living crematory? If you can find anything in Canada to beat that, let me know. I don't think the Patient's death was hastened at all, for I expected her to die that day.

I am sorry poor Miss Bennett had to go through an operation. All to no purpose. Quite possibly she may have Tuberculosis of the kidney.

The man with the Pterygium turned up all right. I removed one the same as Connell did mine, the other I dissected from the cornea and stitched it to conjunctiva of the eyelid. Both have done well. I amputated a finger a few days ago. I had a case of diphtheretic croup, performed Tracheotomy, but of course the child died. Still it was the right thing to do as it was the only chance.

I expect to have to amputate a leg in a week or so. The people are agitating to have a hospital built here and it is very likely to be accomplished. A surgeon will be appointed. I wonder who will get it?

I was at a very nice little party on Friday evening. The programme consisted of music, singing and dancing.

My cousin, Dr. Cross, was up to see me a short time ago. He had a gang of 20 men with him. He owns a lot of land up here. He sold in one day what gave him a profit of $1000. Everything he touches turns to money. He is worth about $100,000 now and he has only been in the colony 10 yrs. When he came here he was abt. $500 in debt. If I could do as well and live long enough, there is not a country or people in the world but what I would see. What is the good of going to heaven ignorant of the earth?

The papers from home last mail contained the sad news that my lovely little native town, Barrie, was nearly flooded to death. Poor thing. I hope it will be able to swim out all right.

I hope you rec. the photos I sent all right. The others will come some time. I have just had my dinner, 6:30 p.m. and I am not going to church as I have to write home, finish your letter, and write a short one to Mr. Fair.

It does seem funny that you should have Miss Herd with you during the holiday. And are she and Grinally throwing mud at each other? They must stop that or they will soon grow out of being in Love. Ask Miss Herd if she remembers the day I drove her and Miss M— from the station when dear old Jack and *Gilly* were going away. She was bound to show her undivided love for Gilly by walking from station to hospital through the mud and rain rather than be found riding in a cab with any other gentleman, but after 2nd thought finally consented. Ask her if she hears from Robinson, the fellow who wanted to take her for a drive 2 days after becoming acquainted. He is better known as (R.P.).

I do wish I were with you, if I wouldn't have fun! I am sure I would put on 10 pounds of fat. People tell me I am looking well as it is. I have gained in flesh a good deal. I must tell you I am taken for 25 — that is the general expression. One lady was so curious as to ask me how old I am. "Oh," I said "I am old enough to be your grandfather." She was abt. 40 & therefore did not believe me. What is the good of telling people your age? Isn't that like a woman? Well, at Allens was the first place I ever refrained from telling my age and the reason I did so then was because Miss A., now Mrs. T., tried by being clever to find out my age, so I fooled her by telling her all sorts of things. They don't know till this day that I am 30. The average Australian young men appear at 23 to be from 29–35. The hot sun during the summer time dries them up. Just fancy, in 5 yrs. more I may look to be 50 or 70, bald headed and wrinkled, ha! ha! what a beautiful picture.

It is winter time and now the fire is going out so I shall have to stop and fire up.

I was consulted by a young lady the other day abt. whiskers. She has a beautiful moustache and a lot of hair on her chin. I made a mash, I know I did. I put on my most sympathetic look and told her the hair on the upper lip rather enhanced than detracted from her beauty, that the Spanish young ladies were proud of such appendages. This young lady is well educated and fairly good looking. So much has this deformity played on her mind that she shuns society, sits in her room and cries. I explained to her that there were not a dozen beings in the world but had something wrong with them sooner or later in life and while she thought she had a terrible affliction 1000's would gladly exchange with her. I explained to her how she was wasting her life by fretting and if she continued to do so, her whole life would be a failure. I advised her to forget herself and try and live for others, to do all the good she could, to make others happy in every way she could and that very soon she would find that she possessed beauty of a very much higher order than ordinary beauty of face. I sent her away happy and have since found a Dr. who can remove the offending hairs by electrolysis. Now after saying all those nice things, don't you think I ought to credit myself with making a mash? Her friends have told me that she is a new girl since that day. I advised her to just have the chin whiskers taken out and leave the moustache.

The agricultural show will be held here on 23 inst. I am told I am put down for judge of something or other, quite likely babies if there is a prize. If so, I shall exhibit that picture and say the little fellow is too ill to come out and thought the picture would do as well.

You remember me telling you I had a patient come 70 miles. Well, she got completely well and another patient came from the same place and is doing well. I charge $5.00 each consultation. I charge double fees for extra work. They think I don't charge enough. Just fancy a patient staying 15 days and just calls once a day at surgery, $75. How would Canadians like such fees? In every case that I examine the urine I charge $5.00. I never do any surgical operation under $5.00. I charged $75. for doing the entropion operation. You may think me an extortioner, but it is the custom of the country, besides, a Dr. who charges high is valued more than a cheap Jack. I just charge the same fees as the best Drs. in Melbourne, if patients don't like it they have the choice of going elsewhere. Poor patients I do not charge, in some cases give rather than take.

It is nearly a year since I left the Old Country. I can scarcely believe it. The time seems to go so fast. Another month and you will be back to your work again. Whatever you do, don't hurt yourself studying. Health is very much easier lost than regained. If your present ailment does not leave you, you must let me prescribe. When I was abt. your age I got all wrong, pale and out of sorts. I prescribed for myself, quit studying and took a sea voyage to Ceylon. I have never regretted it for I have been well ever since with the exception of La Grippe. There is nothing like the sea, the dear old sea, to give a person back their color, to rejuvenate the nerves and give a new lease of life.

I hope you liked the gum leaves to eat, *dear little possum.* When you want any more just let me know and I shall send you some. Your endearing names run like this, "kitten," "porpoise," "Possum." Now which do you really like best?

Whenever you come across a good book in your reading, tell me about it, so that I may read it too.

SCALE OF MEDICAL AND SURGICAL FEES

Comparison of Fees Charged by W.C.L. (1890–93) with Established Rates in Victoria, Australia (c.1893) and Ontario, Canada (1880)

		ONTARIO	VICTORIA	W.C.L.
Ordinary advice or visit within a mile's distance	Day:	$1.00–$2.00	$2.50–$5.00 (10/6 to 1 gn.)	$2.50–$5.00
of practitioner's residence	Night:	$2.00–$5.00	Double	Double for extra work
Ordinary visit at one mile's distance	Day:	$1.50–$2.50	$5.00–$10.00 (1 to 2 gns.)	
	Night:	50%–100% per mile	Double	
Every mile beyond the first	Day:	50ᶜ	$2.50 (10/6)	$1.80 (7/6)
	Night:	50ᶜ–$1.00	$5.00 (1 gn.)	
Midwifery – Natural Labor		$6.00–$10.00	$15.00 & up	$15.00–$30.00
Complicated		$10.00–$20.00		$75.00 including 20 miles at night
Major Obstetric Operations			$250.00–$1,000.00	
Minor Surgery		$10.00–$20.00	$10.00–$25.00	No surgery under $5.00
Tonsilectomy				$10.00–$15.00
Minor Eye Operations			$25.00–$125	$50.00–$75.00
Amputation – Minor		$30.00–$60.00	$25.00–$50.00	
Major		$75.00–$100	$125–$250	$200.00 (arm)
Fractures – Simple		$10.00–$20.00	$25.00–$100	$25.00 (type not specified)
Compound		$15.00–$50.00		
Consultation		$2.00–$10.00	$10.00–$25.00	

Adapted from fee tables in Ludwig Bruck, *The Australasian Medical Directory and Handbook*, Sydney, Bruck, 1892, pp. 33-4 and "Tariff of Fees adopted by the Newcastle and Trent Medical Division of the College of Physicians and Surgeons of Ontario in 1880," reprinted in R.M. Matthews, "Philosophy of the Fee Schedule," *Ontario Medical Review*, Vol.31 (1964), pp. 21-23

Medical fees in Australia (as well as the prices of horses and luxury items) were usually cited in guineas (gns.) rather than pounds (£'s). One guinea equalled one pound plus one shilling (or 21 s., or 21/-); half a guinea was ten shillings and six pence (or 10s. 6d., or 10/6).

Until 1931, the Australian pound was at par with Sterling and was officially worth a little more than $4.86 Canadian. For the sake of convenience, W.C.L. usually converted both pounds and guineas at the rate of 1:5, though he sometimes made allowances for the extra value of the guinea.

I must close with kind regards to Miss Abbott. I was going to say LOVE without any salt, but that wouldn't do, it would spoil. Did you ever notice how easy it is to send Love to a person that you don't care whether they will take it or not, and to those or the one your feelings would like to send it to, you simply can't? Just fancy, give my love to the dog Nero, how absurd, and yet how easy to do.

I look for your letters every mail and if they don't come I think the Boat has gone down. Write me whenever your feelings prompt you to do so. I shall write you next mail.

Yours as always
Wm. C. Little

What do you think of those lines?
Are they getting too close?

Monday August 4th

Dear Possum,

I have just returned from the country. I had a lovely 8 mile ride. The morning is just glorious, everything seems delighted, even the birds are exceptionally happy. My I did ride fast. I have a lovely mare, she has every confidence in me. When I want her to go fast, I clap her on the neck and call, Grace darling. Oh, I did not tell you before that I called her after you. I call her Gracy. Horseback riding is manly sport. I was complimented this morning by a good horseman on the easy way I sat on the saddle. The beauty of riding is to sit up straight and keep quiet in the saddle no matter how fast the horse goes. I wear leggings which come half way up my thighs so that I go fast through mud and water. I waded through the creek, had to hold my feet up to keep them dry.

The patient I was out to see this morning is going out of her head and what to do with her I do not know. I have ordered her to be taken out for a walk in the sun every day to see if old Sol will work a change on her mental functions.

I am just writing this sheet to fill up the letter for it will cost a shilling anyway. So I might as well take the good of it, like you and the Chinese laundry man. If a woman makes a good bargain, how tickled she is.

Now Grace, the next letter I hope to hear of you being quite well, no sore throats. Whoever is treating you, stick to him until he effects a cure.

I wonder if you will be able to read this beautifully painted letter. It's an old daub. I can't write and therefore I won't try to do what I can't do, for that would be failure.

Now Grace, good bye, and may you always be happy.

Sincerely, your W.C.L.

P.S. England and Australia are the only countries that know and thoroughly understand horseback riding.

(Rec. Nov. 3, 1890
Ans. Nov. 5, 1890)

Warracknabeal
Sept. 28, 1890

My dear Grace,

I begin this letter with feelings of disappointment for I have not rec. what you sent me by Dr. Cross. He arrived safely in Sydney over a week ago. I suppose he is so much taken up with the *beauties* of the place that he cannot leave — I mean the scenery, etc. I wish he would send that parcel on for I am curious like a woman to know what is inside of it. The note too, I want to see it. I have written him to come next week as our agricultural show is held here then.

Such a scrubby letter I sent you last mail. Now don't you go thinking I am neglecting you, far from it. The fact was I completely wearied out and could not write. I felt like the disciples [who] when asked to watch, fell asleep. I have had a very pleasant and enjoyable week. My brother has been visiting me since last week. He just came on time for there was a grand ball in the town that evening. I took him and introduced him around to all the ladies and, to judge from appearances, he enjoyed himself very much. About the middle of the evening I was called in consultation over the post-master who took ill very suddenly and was quite unconscious. We decided to trephine[37] the skull, which we did. In the morning, patient died, never for a moment gaining consciousness. We had a P.M. and found an abscess a little below where we had trephined, also abscess of the middle ear.

Trephining is all very well, but it is a good deal speculative. However it is the proper thing to do when you see a patient is going to die, it might save him — a chance — if not, no harm done.

I have had a very quiet week, fortunately, as I have had plenty of time to drive my brother around. I made abt. $15 a day this week. That would be considered good in Canada, don't you think so?

What beautiful weather we are having now. I never saw such lovely days in all my life. The climate for the past month is likely to continue for the next two mos. and is all that heaven could wish to be. Winter is over and just fancy, I was in a garden a few days ago in which the orange trees were covered with ripe oranges. Also, the Lemon trees had plenty of fruit on.

Do you play lawn tennis? I have played a good deal lately. I find the exercise good since I have given up the saddle and taken to the buggy again as the roads are once more good.

By the time you see this you will be back to College again, studying up symptoms, diagnoses, etc. You will find the most difficult of all to make out, viz, "Prognosis," people want to know when their friends are going to die or get better.

I have been lucky enough to prognose several deaths within an hour or two, but in the majority of cases it is a difficult matter to estimate how much life a man has in him as it is not a definite quantity in each. I was called to see a Chinaman Wednesday night. I was asked if the patient was bad. I said yes, that he would die. The friends wanted to know when. Well, I said, if he were an Englishman he couldn't live more than six hours and that I couldn't be sure how long a Chinaman would live, particularly as he was soaked with opium. Poor Chinamen think I know everything. The Chinaman died in 4 hours.

Yes, the great mistake in medical teaching is students are too much lectured at and not nearly enough bedside clinics. Anything I know about death and its signs I have had to pick up as I go along. There are many points which might be brought under the student's notice that would help him very much indeed.

I am beginning to get a little proud of my treatment of phthisis. I have had what I consider wonderful results, no one more surprised than myself. I give you two formulae I use and which I have improved since I mentioned it [sic] to you before.

You may have the opportunity of trying those mixtures. [38] If so, give them a good trial and I think you will be greatly pleased. One case in particular I feel elated over was in the person of a Bank clerk who was simply dying, both the apices of the lungs gone. Temp. 102, had failed to a skeleton. I gave him No. 2 with Liq. pepticus, Liq. Arsenicalis chlor. and acid hydrochlor to be taken after meals. The results were simply astonishing. The poor fellow has gained in flesh and spirits. No doubt he will not last a year but a life prolonged 6 mos. or a year is sometimes very important. I shall tell you more about this young man in the future.

Well, Grace, I had a long talk to my brother last night, relating experiences. I must say he has had as variable experience as I ever had. How funny that we should both have such roving dispositions. My brother was criticizing the Menagerie and I think you are a bit too deep for him. "Blame it all," he said "I think she would know too much." I laughed and said, "Would you like to read a letter from [her]?" "Yes," he said, he would be delighted. So I read the one with the description of your bedroom in and so on, etc. What do you think he said? I don't know that I should tell you. "Well," he said "She *is* a nice innocent girl and learning has not spoiled her." I told him all about the good times we had at 40 Stewart St., the scrapes I got into, the mesmerism racket, which tickled him very much. I thought he would have hurt himself laughing when I told him abt. the Napanee expedition. I laugh over that affair yet, when the ridiculousness of the thing strikes me. I wish I could have some of the good old times over again. You know I have to be so here, always the Dr. I am getting accustomed to it now, but for a time at first I felt in harness a bit. I suppose the reason was I was a little old before being broken in. There is lots of room to act a little, but I hear you say acting is sham. Well, just come into my surgery as a patient and see if I am natural or not. I do feel and act differently with a man when he is a patient than if I meet him under other circumstances. I can't help it.

My brother took me down a peg last week. I rather fancied myself as a billiard player so I challenged him to play 10 games for a $1.50, I to give him 25 points in 50. We only required to play 6 games for he won 5 and I won one. So I lost the money. It served me right. I should not have been so conceited. You must not think me a chronic gambler, I bet occasionally just for the fun of it. One night at a billiard tournament one player was a good deal ahead of the other. A rather pompous fellow appeared to wager 2–1 on the man who was ahead. I immediately took him up. The man who was behind, a friend of mine, took courage and beat the man who was leading. I won $5.00. A few nights afterwards the same pompous fellow offered the same bet and I took him up and won $2.50. He says now he won't bet with me anymore as I always change the luck. Now, Grace, you must not think me a wicked man betting like that. There is no possible danger of me becoming a chronic gambler. I just fancy if you had been in my place you would have bet against that fellow. I don't know how it is but at times the very devil gets into me, which makes me a little reckless. Then I settle down and be good again. Australia is a great sporting country, all kinds of sports. I am getting to like Australia much better than Canada. I think there is more get up in the people in this country, i.e., in some respects only. The Canadian Women are far superior to the Australians. There is not that modesty amongst the ladies of this country that is found in Canada. There is a certain amt. of looseness and what I would term vulgarity, which I do not like. Possibly I may become accustomed to it, but I hope not.

By the way, I made a very funny discovery the other day. While in the Bank in conversation with the teller, Mr. Bell, I recognized him to be a Scotch man. I asked him what part of Scotland he came from and found out he came from where my relatives live and that he is a distant relation of mine. Isn't that strange? I thought there was some affinity between us, for I had taken quite a liking to him. I have no end of relations. I find I have a cousin in New Zealand and if I ever go to the North Pole I may find some there.

I have just stopped for a while and reread yours of July 14. You might tell me about Miss Herd & Dr. Gilles. I can quite understand if they crossed swords or any misunderstanding arose between them, it would not be easy to make it up again, for Dr. G. is an unrelenting, unforgiving man.

My brother is bothering me to send a message to you, so here it goes. If you are as good a dr. as you look cute in that Menagerie picture you would be very foolish to practise in Canada; that if you decide to come out here he will hunt up a good practice for you in one of the cities. The only consideration he asks in return is that if he takes ill you will have to attend him free. (Eratum — cute should read charming.) I have no doubt he would send a great deal more, but I won't let him.

I have just been stopped for a while by two calls, one a woman who apparently is going wrong in her mind. I did not tell the husband what I thought. I will try treatment for a while. Besides, it is not good practice to tell patients every time what is the matter. The other call is to attend a minister's wife in confinement. It won't be necessary to see her for a few hours yet, so I shall finish this letter.

One of my patients the other day presented me with a live Swan. You are fond of pets. I would send it to you if I could.

So you are going to the Old Country with your mother and brother. That will be real nice. I know you will enjoy London so much. Go to all the theatres just to see how Londoners spend their evenings. I wish I were there, I would try and persuade you to let me take you around and give you an insight into the — at least some of the — mysteries of London. Wouldn't you come? I fancy you would for you, like myself, are a little curious. These things are all right so long as a person's head is screwed on properly. You will have a hard winter's work, but remember my sage advice, don't work too hard or you will become *anaemic* and that would spoil your looks. It is much easier to lose good blood than to get it back. I often think it is even more important for a woman to religiously look to her health than a man. I never write the word woman in a letter to you but I think of the day I said "My dear woman" and you got quite vexed. I saw I put my foot in it. I could always read your feelings; I could feel the reproof even if you did not utter it. I give you still the same credit I did in Kingston of having more influence over me than any other *girl* I ever met. I was nearly going to write "woman," but I think you will not object to "girl," "lady" is so formal. If I could write as I would talk, how much easier it would be to write letters. I always think, well, someone else may read the letter and how foolish it would appear. There is one thing I have partly told you and which, whenever I think of it, makes me feel rather little of myself, and that is abt. the time I was in Lachute. I felt somewhat strange: I don't know whether you noticed it or not. I fancy you did. You know I am a very independent fellow, at least I feel that way, and far too much for my own good. Well, I did not rec. your letter inviting me to Lachute, I only rec. the postal card. Well, to tell you the truth, at the time I thought it a little cool and that you were not very particular whether you saw me again or not. Wasn't I a fool after you sending me such a nice letter, but I did not get it. Didn't you think me a little distant?

I have just returned from attending the case I mentioned. I went to church, was sitting in front seat, church packed full, when I was called. It is the first time I have been called out of church. Well, it is a boy and the Baptist Minister is delighted for the other two are girls. Babies are wonderful institutions, most interesting so long as there are not too many of them.

I have not had my picture taken yet. I am about buying another pair of horses, so I shall have myself, horses and buggie taken and will send the results to you. I shall be delighted, Grace, if you get that model taken and send it to me. I just mention it this time so you won't forget. I have made up my mind to get one, either model or hand, which will you give? I leave you to guess which I would like best. I have a beautiful garden. I shall pluck a flower and send it to you. I suppose it won't look much by the time it has travelled 12,000 miles.

Well, I have nearly chewed the rag all to pieces so will have to wind up. I would rather chew the rag with you while sitting in the chair that goes "Creak, Creak" for two hours than write a 100-page letter.

How is Miss Abbott? Give her my kind regards and tell her if ever she comes to Australia, to come and see me. Remember me to Miss Herd and ask her how her "Spinal Column" is.

I have not heard from Shuttleworth since I left. I wrote him a long letter, which he may not have received. My father has sold the farm and is going to live in Toronto. When I get the Toronto address I shall give it to you so that you may call the next time you are in Toronto. My sister Maggie would like to meet you for she says she knows by your picture you are a nice girl. I think you would like Maggie a good deal.

How is Mrs. Savage and the boy? Does he wear pants yet?

Well, this is a pretty long letter and should in a measure make up for the last.

Now, good-bye, Opossum, and remember I am delighted to hear from you. Your letters add a bright thread to the web of my life.

I am as ever,

Your sincere   ————————   Wm. C. Little

(Rec. Nov. 28, 1890
Ans. Nov. 30, 1890)

Warracknabeal
Oct. 26, 1890

My dear Grace,

I am so sorry, I have run out of your paper. I have to write you on this slippery stuff as the heavy paper would cost too much.

I received your two last letters both together so I had a feast. They were two very different letters, one quite yourself and the other as if you were out of humor. However I don't mind you being out of humor, for when you get back into it again you are very good.

First of all, I must thank you for that (well, my brother called it the missing link) paper weight. I do laugh at the blamed thing, the way it stares and grins at a person. I must tell you the fun I had with it. I have a melancholic patient, very serious, thinks she is going out of her head. She always gives me the blues and I wish her far enough. She came to see me a few nights after I got the "Missing Link" and she was so gloomy, I placed the "Missing Link" on the table before her so that the light shone on *its* face. "Now," I said, "I want you to stare at that thing until it makes you laugh." Great United States! — she went into fits of laughter, the first laugh she had had for four months. I sent her home without giving her medicine and told her that from this time forth I would put her under the care of the Missing Link. I charged 10/6 all the same.

Dr. Cross[39] spent a week with me. I did enjoy his visit very much. I kept him pretty busy all the time. I fancy Cross must have told you some outlandish yarns. If he told you all he said he did, I don't wonder at your thinking him cheeky. I told him you considered he had a considerable [cheek]. He is about getting a practice with a hospital appointment attached. If he gets it, it will be a good thing.

I have been very busy during the past three weeks, one week I did not get more than 12 hrs. sleep altogether. I was nearly tired out. I made $125 one day. The other Dr. who was here went out of his mind and had to be put in an asylum. I told you about his wife's death some time ago. I think he was addicted to morphia; in fact I am sure of it.

There is a Dr. doing Locum Tenens for him and another Dr. has settled here. I feel all right no matter how many come. I am doing all the work. I prescribed for 22 patients yesterday besides my own town visits, which amounted to 32 or £16 or $80. The other two had only one patient between them. I don't know which one got *it*. This is an anxious time for me now for there is one Dr. I want to keep out of here as he practised here before and was well liked, so I naturally don't want to see him back again as he might stand a better chance of the hospital appointment than I would. The Dr. who is doing Locum Tenens is a very fine fellow and I wish he would stay. We would then combine to run No. 3 out as he is not required. That would be right, would it not?

I was so sorry to learn that Dr. Irwin departed this life so suddenly. I wonder did he know he had an aneurysm. If I had one I would not want to know about it for I would always be thinking the thing would go off bang. I had a letter from Mr. Fair last mail. He is tickled to death over that baby, that wonderful baby, and also over the prospects of another one. It is astonishing how some men like babies. There is an old crank here who has 16 of a family and, no matter where you meet him, he will begin and yarn abt. those 16 brats. I have seem some of them and they are as ugly as sin, cross-eyed, etc.

Poor Miss Bennett has become a somnambulist. I wouldn't wonder if she will turn out a regular hypnotist, magnetizer, etc. She certainly acts strangely. Oh, by the way, you want to know what I meant by that sentence. Well, you know I was deeply in *love* with her and she would not love me in return, not even a little bit and — ha, ha, ha, ha. How strangely funny. Well, what I really meant was that Miss Bennett never acted the same when I was present as when absent. She was two girls in one in other words; had she been her real self with me we would have been good friends whereas we parted entire strangers. I believe from what you say she may go wrong in her mind or become a very wonderful person, magnetically and nervously, and be able to read minds as well as your humble servant!

I met a clever mind reader last night. He could tell me what I was thinking about by simply holding my hand. I can read minds pretty well but not so well as that. To read a mind well, I must either be in love or hate, two extremes. You remember I could read your mind pretty well. Did you ever try to make a person turn around who was walking ahead of you. I have, and when feeling magnetically, I have often done it successfully three or four times while the medium was walking a short distance. I have often tried it in R.R. cars with like results. I am going to give some attention to hypnotism for I believe it can be used with advantage in treating nervous diseases.

You ask me what my honest opinion of Dr. G. is. Well, I have a kindly feeling for poor old Gilly, but my honest opinion always was that he would sacrifice his best friend to accomplish his ends. I would not trust him implicitly, always beware and on guard. Sly old Gilly I always called him. I liked G. in many things. He had some very strong traits in his character, which I admire wherever found and no matter what the combination. One day while G. and I were having a quiet talk in the park he nearly cried when speaking of his mother and sister and how he had been estranged from home. His life has been one continuous fight against opposition, every step that he advanced was by plodding and hard work. He has a peculiar mixture of love and hate in his character. I admired G. for the many good points in his character and overlooked the weaker ones, knowing that he had not the privileges that many other young men had.

Miss H[erd], if she has fallen out with G., will not speak well of him. Dr. F. is a genuine fellow, everything done fair and above board. A man I would trust. I shall get all G.'s doings from Dr. Jack some time. I think I have answered all your questions.

So, you have made your mind up to wear a bonnet next spring. For goodness' sake send me your photo until I see how you look. If you get a nice little one, all right, but if you get an old woman's one you will look horrid. Just fancy a big thing coming down over your ears and away down the back of your neck with strings down to the ground.

I am just wondering what to get you for a Xmas present. It is so far to send anything. I know what I would get you were I in Montreal, another dark red dress the same as the one you wore at 40 Stewart St.

What do you call that dress, morning gown? I shall never forget the morning you kept facing me and trying to attract my attention so that I wouldn't notice the absence of ——.

By the way, one of my patients who is on his death bed willed me a valuable horse worth abt. $180, pretty good isn't it? The Dr's. bill will be as much more. I don't know why he did so unless he considered I have been very attentive to him. Poor man, I am sorry for him, he has phthisis and is sinking fast. He does look so pleased when I call to see him. His spirits always keep up for abt. 4 hours after my visit. He is engaged to be married and was looking forward to his marriage day with bright hopes, but they are all gone now. His young lady comes and nurses him every day, which pleases him very much. The hands of love can do things so much better than any other.

I have a lot of bad cases now, which worry me a good deal. I have a diphtheria patient in my house and no one in the town knows about it. Two children in the family died of it during the past few weeks and the only daughter, aged 15, has it very bad. They lived so far from the town that it was impossible for me to go out often. The father was nearly frantic about the daughter and wanted to leave her in the town in order that I might see her as often as required but no one would take her in. The father came to me crying so I took pity on him and took her in and am happy to say she is nearly well now. I send her home tomorrow. She had diphtheria of the nose as well as throat. Not a soul in the town knows anything about it. I told the father if he mentioned it to a soul I would have her sent away. If my patients knew abt. it they would not come near me. I am careful to wash my hands and change my coat etc. before I visit them.

I noticed what you said abt. the French boy. I think it was real kind of you to look after him when he was in the hands of a lot of ignorant Frenchies.

I must close now for want of time. Next letter will be longer, I promise, and probably more sensible. I have to write home yet. So good bye and as ever I remain your sincere friend.

Wm. C. Little

P.S. The flower I sent you was a broken heart or something about the heart. I don't know exactly (Mitral Stenosis, I think).

I have a beautiful *garden.*

(Rec. Dec. 29th, 1890
Ans. Jan. lst, 1891)

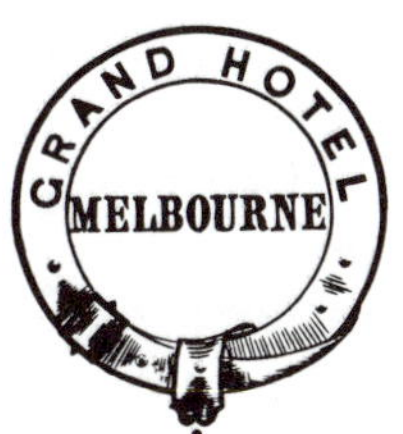

Grand Hotel
Melbourne, Nov. 25th, 1890

My dear Grace

You will see by the address that I am not at home. How funny to call a place out here "home." Well, I am in Melbourne having a rest. I prescribed for myself on this occasion. The fact of the matter is, I was simply killing myself and I did not know it until it just dawned upon my mind that I was not feeling like myself a bit. "Busy" is not strong enough to let you know how much practice I have been doing during the past 5 or 6 months. I became fearfully nervous, could not sleep and when I would just doze off, I would suddenly start. Dr. Cross came to my assistance in a most opportune time. Holidays, holidays, glorious holidays, and how I am enjoying them. My nerves are quieting down and I am beginning to feel quite myself again. I am simply dissipating in a mild way. I go to theatres, operas, races, anything to completely turn my mind from practice and patients. I am just going to take a short sea voyage for the good of my appetite. I have spent a pleasant time in Ballarat and Geelong, both of which places I send you views of. It will give you some idea of what I am seeing. I have visited some of the gold mines. Geelong is a nice quiet place situated on the sea coast. The air is fresh and bracing and the scenery, well, fairly charming. When I was in Ballarat my brother came in on me quite unexpectedly, so I made him take a holiday with me. Of course I pay the shot. My holiday trip will cost me more than it would to go home via England. Everything is very expensive out here.

Billy Brown, whom you have heard me speak abt., has just come in and wants to know who I am writing to. I have just said to a nice little porpoise out in the sea.

I received your last letter of Oct. 6th, which date a year ago I sailed from Southampton for Australia. You appear to be quite happy in your new quarters and it must be exciting having to attend lectures with such a large proportion of the male element. I am glad you have recovered from your illness. Don't get nervous like me.

Yes, the letter you received from me was a mean little grumbly thing. I was just beginning to get run down then. It is awfully hard to write a whole souled letter sometimes, isn't it? Do you know, I fancy you do, that I cannot write you as good a letter now as I could a year ago and why, I wonder. Well, because I have not been in your company for such a long time. I would require to go back to Canada and get charged with magnetism again and if it were not so far I would go, but oh me, I have to stick here. Well, where am I drifting to? I think what I want to say is that letters at best are dry things compared with a personal interview. There are the many little things which occur day by day which help to make life pleasant and at the same time bring out the best that is in a man.

I have just been stopped for a while to listen to some of Billy Brown's love stories, which are many and very innocent. He doesn't know how it is but when he meets a young lady and she is nice to him he cannot help it and so falls in love. I have had so many laughs at him. He says it is not his fault, the girls string him on and he just falls in love to please them.

A funny thing occurred yesterday while I was in conversation with a gentleman in this hotel. I happened to be standing at the door when lo and behold a young Canadian who lives 16 miles from my home passed by. I hailed him, well, he was quite surprised. He is looking after the interests of his father's reaper and binder firm. He is making lots of money. I think he is going home in about a month. If so, I shall send you something which he will mail to you.

By the way, there is a lady Dr. practising in Melbourne. I called on her a few days ago to know how a patient I had sent her was getting on. It was the young woman with the whiskers. Well, they have all been removed, much to the young lady's joy. Dr. Constance Stone[40] studied in Toronto and of course knew people I knew. She is real nice and in possession of a fair amount of good looks. It is funny how I get on with the lady Meds., isn't it?

I have been doing a little special work on the eye with the best man here. He is so nice and he and I can hit it together nicely. He will assist me by letter with any cases I may require advice on. I am in with the best men here, which may be to my advantage some day.

Now I must take Mr. Brown to dinner and hear more about his loves.

Dinner is over and I have returned from a stroll in the gardens. Oh, I sent you some papers, in one of which you will see a garden scene by gas light. I laughed when I saw it, as it reminded me of an innocent remark you made abt. spooning going on all over the world. I believe you are right. I went to the wax works one evening in company with a very fine English Dr. One part of the building is occupied by a fortune teller with a big round painted face, low-necked dress and short skirts. A horrid looking creature. She was so vulgarly ugly that I decided to have my fortune told. She tells fortunes by cards. She began by asking me questions. I informed her that I came to have my fortune told, not to answer questions. I cut the cards 3 times. The funny part of it is, she told me 9/10 which was true. She told me I was in competition with a dark-haired gentleman abt. business matters, that he was doing his best to beat me but I would win. Since the other Dr. at Warracknabeal went insane, the government appointments are vacant. Another dark-haired Dr. is doing his level best to get them. The Health Officership is granted by the Shire Council. This Dr. had secured 3 of the leading men in the council to vote for him and had said he was sure of the appointment. Being a new chum, I was a little slow, but fast enough to beat him. I got 9 votes and he got only 3. The Public vaccinator has to be appointed and I find he has been down here trying his best to get it. I at once secured the service of the local M.P. to work for me. The result will be known on Tuesday. He was nearly getting the appointment when my MP stepped in. The Appointments are worth $500 a year. This ugly witch told me a great deal of stuff that was quite true and a lot of lies. She said my life had been lucky and would continue to be so, that I would get married and that my wife would die first (I wonder if that will come true), and I would not marry again. Now what do you think of my fortune? Oh, I am to be rich some day & I will travel a great deal. Talk about luck! I spent an evening with an American dentist in Ballarat — a card party at which we played for money. I won $8. Now, you must not think me a gambler, no, no, I am not. I make myself agreeable at a card party and if small stakes are on, why I do the same, not caring a cent whether I win or lose. I know you won't like it but if you knew the circumstances you would feel the same as I do about it.

I was at a grand bicycle tournament yesterday; I got wildly excited. My English Dr. friend was with me. There are more sports in this country in one month than in Canada in 12.

A friend has called so I shall finish this in the evening.

Monday Morning

I am feeling grand this morning. I rec. a letter from Cross saying he is making me abt. $50 a day and that he can stay two weeks longer if I wish. Isn't it too bad that I am so far from Montreal? I would be so delighted to see you and give you a grind on [the] practice of Med. You should know pneumonia pretty well. If I were in Montreal I could buy you that gown like the one I liked. If I only had the model [of your hand] I would send you a pair of gloves. You see I don't know your size. You might give me the size & sometime when I take the notion you might get a pair of kangaroo gloves. I had kangaroo tail soup the other night and it makes me feel like jumping! This is a very nice country and I want you to see it and let me make the plan for you to see it. When you go back to England it will be a very simple matter to go back to Canada via Australia and if you have your mother with you, you need not be afraid of getting lost. I will look after you while here, will show you all the beauties of Australia & Tasmania and, of course, will pay expenses. If you cannot prevail on your mother to come, why not try and steal Mrs. Savage away? She is such good company. Now don't let Mr. Savage see this or I am as good as dead. Don't you think so? One year from now we have this trip. What say you?

Remember me to Miss Abbott.

I remain your sincere ——————   Wm. C. Little
                                    (No rulers required this time.)

P.S. It is raining very hard. I think I am some kind of a water animal, Devil fish probably, for I always love wet weather.

P.P.S. If you are ever in Toronto, call at 49 Grant St. as my Father & Mother & sisters have gone to the city to live. Now be sure & call & see them.

(Rec. Jan. 24, 91
Ans. Jan. 25, 91)

Warracknabeal
Dec. 22, 1890

My dear Grace,

I rec. your welcome letter of Nov. 5th just 3 days ago. I was very glad to hear from you as your letters, of all Canadian letters, are so refreshing.

When I wrote you last I was taking a holiday. Well, that is over now and I have returned to practice again feeling a new man altogether. Some poet has said,
> "The sweet vicissitudes of rest & toil
> Make labour easy and renew the soil."

I feel renewed. I could jump over a stake and railed fence without touching the top rail. That's pretty good for an old man, isn't it?

What do you think, I am called the old Dr. now. Just fancy! I feel quite big about it, — ha! ha! The old Dr., the man of Experience, the old reliable, great Heavens! It makes me smile in my shoes and fancy I am some old family man, an Elder in the church with one of my sons — the oldest boy, singing in the choir. Well, I like the name "old Dr." anyway, and to keep it up I am going to start to pull my hair out, to get bald, for it is inclined to be thicker than when in Canada.

This is a great country for hair. I examined a man a few days ago for insurance and he had a mane down his back like a horse, he was a funny specimen, half baboon, I think.

Poor Dr. Cross was nearly killed with work when he was here. He made me $600 in three weeks, which was not bad. He thinks I have struck a Gold Mine. Cross has settled about 35 miles from me. He will make about $4500 a year.

Well, Grace, I have a new opposition here. I don't know how we will get along together. While I was away, he got one of my patients. I had been engaged to attend the woman in confinement; while I was away she took a bit ill and sent for Dr. G. [R.H. Gibbs]. By some means he got the case, but as luck would have it, he got stuck in the job and had to send for me. I gave the husband the d—— about having the young Dr. to attend a case I was engaged for. I had to deliver the woman, much to the chagrin of Dr. G. I charged the man $25 for his cheek and told him it served him right.

This young dr. is a bit chicken hearted, but will do anything to get a patient from me, which I don't care a bit, but it is the way he does it. I was called in consultation with him a week ago, a case of Empyema. I recommended operation. So he wanted to know when. I suggested right away. When it came to the time, he took up the chloroform bottle and said, "Oh, you operate." I said it was his case and he should operate. He was very nervous. I cut down in the child's chest and got ½ pint pus out, much to the delight of the parents. I wouldn't let another Dr. operate on a case of mine, even if I knew he could do it a little better than myself.

I had a letter from Mr. Fair last mail which made me laugh. He is the happy father of another daughter and he blames me for bringing it into the world 2 wks. too soon. He had just rec. a letter from me and there happened to be a very ridiculous sentence in it which he nearly killed himself laughing over. He showed it to Mrs. Fair and she went into convulsions of laughter, which were immediately followed by labor pains. K.N. Fenwick will begin to think my F.O.S. is better than his since I can influence labor 15,000 miles away. Funny thing, wasn't it?

I really do not know what sentence you refer to that you cannot make out. Letters are very confusing sometimes, particularly if you write faster than you think or think faster than you write. In a letter you cannot get the expression on the countenance so that what may be penned in earnest may be considered a joke or otherwise. Now Grace, supposing — I can never write that without smiling. I think of your engineer or cowboy away in Texas without money but fearfully much in love. Well, supposing we, just for fun, write a letter to each other, a regular long one and put everything in it we think of, say for one day, let it be good, bad or indifferent. The letters to be written on the same day and when read, burned. What a crazy idea, but do you know I have often thought what a fascinating novel such an one would be. I fear none would be game to do it. I will never improve in my writing or English. I am more of the mechanical turn of mind than literary.

Well, I have to stop and go and attend a confinement.

Monday Morning

I have been busy all morning and consequently have only ¾ of an hr. to finish this letter. I am sending you one or two papers, Xmas numbers, they are not very much — not so good as "Montreal Herald."

I was flattered this morning by a patient coming 60 miles to see me. I would practise a good while in Canada before I would be known 60 & 80 miles from the town. I am in love with my practice and well I might be, for I am sure there are not 10 other Drs. in Australia that do more and not two in Canada. For instance this morning I have had a

Fracture	$25.00
Excision of tonsils	$10.00
Above patient 60 miles	$ 5.00
Sprained elbow	$ 5.00
Two consultations	$ 5.00
	$50.00

Well, that looks like blowing my own horn, but I don't mean it. It is merely drawing a comparison between Australian and Canadian practice.

I have a busy month ahead of me as I am engaged to attend 18 confinements. I hope they all don't happen on the same day.

So you like Montreal better than Kingston. I am sure you see five times more practical work at any rate, and that is what stands good in practice. What a confidence it gives you when called to a case and you have seen any amt. of similar cases. You know what to do and how to do it.

Now Grace, don't become all in all a Dr. or it will spoil you. I much prefer to think of you as you were at 40 Stewart St., a good deal for innocent fun and not very terribly anxious to kill yourself studying, than to think of you as a clever Dr. Do you understand me rightly I wonder? I have and always will feel that it is possible for a girl studying a profession in which the feelings must be kept in subjection, to be able to look on the most blood-curdling sights without showing any external emotion, to become cold and possibly stern, qualities which are never admired in a woman. I don't think there is any fear of you degenerating in that way, is there?

I do not know what has happened to Shuttleworth. He has never written me. I am quite put out with him. Can you tell me if he graduated last spring?[41]

Do you know Dr. Nichol in Montreal? I met his son, also a Dr. Nichol, while in Edinburgh. You may remember me introducing him to you at Reunion. If you meet him kindly remember me to him.

We are having the most delightful weather now, not a bit like last year. It seems so funny to think you have snow and ice at home while here the farmers are busy taking off the wheat. By the way, we had a regular hail storm last week. It simply came down in chunks, the only natural ice I have seen since I left Canada. I am reading Mark Twain's "In the Court of King Arthur." Some parts of it are very amusing.

I try to get an hour's reading every day and also an hour to study my cases. I believe I could give you a pretty good grind now. Do you know anything of Graves' disease?[42] I have three cases. They are very interesting cases as there is such a diversity of symptoms.

Well, I haven't got you that gown yet. Just keep patient and you may get it some day. All things come to those who wait — like the model I am still waiting [for]. Did I say I must have the model or the hand? I may have said that. If so, all I can say is that it was a bit cheeky. I am getting more cheeky I believe. I don't blush now — at least very seldom. You know it was you that made me blush so much at 40 [Stewart St.]. Well, I am not so sensitive now, it wouldn't do in this hot country. What a mixed up letter, but I shall send it knowing you will forgive all that is not just right.

Your sincere   Wm. C. Little

I am the bottom line, just a bit ahead of you, ha, ha.

(Rec. Feb. 21, 91
Ans. do.)

Warracknabeal
Jan. 18, 1891

My dear Grace,

Here I am cooped up in the surgery, doors & windows shut, the temp. abt. 100, the wind blowing clouds of dust which finds its way into the house through the slightest crack. I am dressed in lawn tennis suit, which makes me look cool whether I feel so or not. However, I must not grumble for we have had a most pleasant summer, beautifully cool, the evenings all anyone could wish for. At any rate I feel that I should be thankful, for I never felt better in all my life & although I never looked well at any time, I think I never looked better than at present. My sad and somewhat grumbly letter from Melbourne would quite likely lead you to think me a mere wreck of my former self. I am quite stout now — in fact, I am *fat,* filling my clothes out ever so much better than I did two months ago. If a girl were to write that wouldn't it sound funny? What an idea, it just came without being asked. I think I shall just write whatever comes into my head and if I do, you know the stipulation — *To be burned at once.* Now do you agree to that or not? Well, I shall wait your answer.

I received your letter of Nov. 30 with the little calendar in it! I was so glad to hear from you. I believe you were more like yourself in this letter than some of the others. I must not criticise as it always stirs up little angry feelings and makes a person want to fight and don't know who to fight with. The ''Ladies' Journal'' is quite interesting, the pictures beautiful. I love to see Elizabeth lying in the water at the foot of the garden, drowned. How peaceful she looks, all her troubles at an end. Suicide in its legal aspect is a horrible thing, but in the tragic and romantic world it often just seems the proper thing, causing a sensational termination. The picture where Joan shivered at the sound of kisses is almost funny. Sounds we are accustomed to don't alarm us. Joan must have been quite a stranger to the sound of kisses or she would not have shivered.

The Queen of the Roses I admired very much, especially the hands, arms and attitude.

You interested me a bit in the French lady student.[43] She must be interesting, in fact I would just love to hear her experience. Fancy her setting

A little girl, aged about 6 years, the daughter of Mr. G. Blythman, of Brim, was brought in to Dr. Little on Wednesday suffering from a fracture of the outer bone of the forearm caused by falling off some bags on a waggon on which she had been playing. On Thursday a boy aged 7½ years, the son of Mr. Gill, of Bangerang, met with an accident. Whilst in the act of jumping from a trap to open a gate he tripped and fell out causing Colles of the wrist. He was attended by Dr. Little. Both patients are doing well.

A workman at Messrs. Rawling and Co's. implement factory met with a painful accident on Monday whilst working the drilling machine. By some means, which he is unable to explain, he overbalanced and fell against the machine, his nose coming in contact with the cogs and being very severely lacerated. Dr. Little was called in and stitched the wound and the injured feature is now healing satisfactorily.

A serious accident happened on Tuesday to a youth named Walter Simpson, aged 17 years. He was in the act of removing the nosebag off his horse, when the animal without warning reared and bolted, striking Simpson on the head with his fore-foot and inflicting a cut 4½in. in length, throwing back the skin from the bone about 2in., and severing three arteries from which blood flowed freely. Dr. Little was immediately called in and tied up the arteries and stitched the wound. The patient is progressing satisfactorily.

"I had a host of accidents Xmas week, some of which you will see mentioned in a paper I sent you . . ."

fractures, reducing dislocations. The resident Dr. must have felt pretty torn over it. Either the Dr. or the people were fools. It is astonishing how credulous the public is. If quackery were allowed full swing, the quack would make more money than the Dr. People imagine a quack is never born and what he can't cure is incurable. Educated people who should know better run after the quack, ministers, lawyers and a hoard of others. Probably if the truth were known about this clever French girl, it would be found that she did the work for ½ the money the Dr. would have done it for.

A very clever nurse came here about 10 days ago. Clever because she says she is. Well, she made herself so *busy* as to solicit the attendance on her own account of a confinement I am engaged to attend. She explained how clever she was, what miracles she had performed, etc. This clever dame called on me a few evenings ago with certificates from ministers and women. I then got her to tell me how clever she was, etc. I quizzed her for about

5 minutes, what she would do in complications. She neither understood what they were nor what to do. I then told her she had better learn those things before she tried to take patients from *me.*

Well, how did the Empyema case get on and what was the treatment? I have had three cases which I operated on and all recovered.

I had a host of accidents Xmas week, some of which you will see mentioned in a paper I sent you, if you get it.

I am getting along very nicely here. At a meeting of the Subscribers to the Hospital I was elected Senior Honorary Medical Officer and an Honorary Surgeon. I was also nominated for committee man, with the result that I pulled as many votes as the highest, both being equal.

So far I think I have landed on my feet coming here. I have another opposition here, but he will not do me any harm as he is either drunk or under the influence of morphia all the time. He has been here a month and has had only one patient.

I feel sorry for the man. I told him when he came he would not do anything as two Drs. could do all the work and that I certainly would give no encouragement to a third.

Well, Grace, by the time you rec. this you will be over your eyes in work. You will have fully realized what a heavy year the final is. I wish I were there to talk and keep you off your work. You know I spent a good deal of time in my final year that was not devoted to study, but then I made up for it by being fresh and more absorptive. You will find genuine study begins with practice. I am getting my book knowledge arranged in a more practical form and I feel I know 20 times more now than when I graduated.

Don't hurt yourself trying to get the work up too well. Before you hear from me again you will be through with examinations. You have my warmest sympathy and best wishes during exam time, and also my perfect confidence that you will be as successful as you have always been. Don't forget my advice about the orals. Put on your most warming smile, be cheerful and confident, and you will surround the examiner with an element that will certainly bring him in sympathy with you. What an influence a plea-sant face has, it makes everything look bright.

I must tell you about an afternoon tea. I had no less than six ladies to afternoon tea last week — one a young married lady who acted as chaperone. Two of the young ladies were from Melbourne, one of them quite interesting, in fact, the only interesting young lady I have met since I came here. She is a Jewess, good looking and accomplished. Well, I showed them the Journal you sent and how learnedly I talked about the latest fashions. I took, or went out, with this Jewess for horseback rides three times. We did a little racing and jumping over logs etc. I must tell you that old dame rumor came and told me she considered I was the *nicest* gentleman in W'Beal. How flattered I should feel. I really don't know for sure whether I swallowed it or not, but I am inclined to think I did — Men are so soft, ain't they? That old dame rumor says that it is regretted in the town that I am engaged. I must tell you about it. I told Mr. Brown for a purpose and in good faith that I am engaged to a young lady in Canada and that I will be married in 2 or 3 years and that said young lady is enormously wealthy. I knew he would go and tell it even [though] he promised not to do so. The result was that it spread like wild fire and it is now generally understood that I am *not* in the market. You see it gives me a better standing as a Dr., for if I am not married I am next thing to it. It had the desired effect, for if I am seen in co. with young ladies, that old Mother Grundy says very little and I go on quite as I want to.

You ask me what I would think if you get converted.[44] Well, I would not think any the less of you, I am sure. I really like to think that my sisters are converted and the same should apply elsewhere.

I fear I am rather materialistic in my views. I am fully satisfied that what is beyond this life is not known by anyone. What is taught may be in good faith, but it is speculative. At present I feel if I make the best possible use of my life here, that I shall have no concern about what is to follow. If I can exist outside this body, then I feel that the best part of life is to come. I shall go on exploring expeditions to the moon and other worlds. As for a hell beyond, such teaching is damnable and could only be concocted by persons of the most cruel turn of mind. Charity is the most beautiful word in the bible. There is no limit to its meaning.

I had a letter from my sister Susie last mail and she asked me to invite you to call anytime you are in Toronto. Address 49 Grant Street. I am sure they will make you very welcome and if I were there you would be doubly so.

Well, I shall have to bring this rambling letter to a close with the promise that tomorrow morning I may add a few more lines if anything new strikes me as being at all interesting to you. I am negotiating about buying a property here at $2500 cash. The only thing that leaves me undecided is the possibility that I may not stay here many years. It is quite probable that I can make as good use of my life here as elsewhere. This place is lacking in Society, a lack I feel very much. I like to improve myself socially

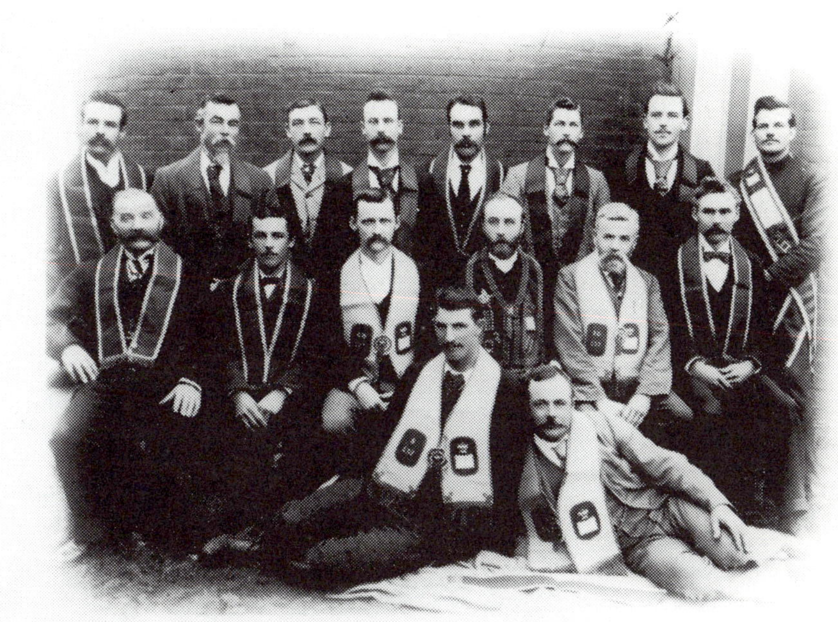

Members of the Warracknabeal Loyal Orange Lodge circa 1895
Dr. Little is third from left in back row

and every other way, but it is mighty hard where the great current runs the other way. I think you would have a great many new shoots to trim off if you were to meet me now. I wonder if they will be grown into big limbs by the time you see me again. It will require an axe and a cross-cut saw to remove them.

I must go to bed so good night — and good morning when you get up.

Jan. 19, 12:15 p.m.

I have been busy all morning so have not much time left until mail closes. I fancy our letters must cross each other in Toronto or somewhere near Montreal. If I write a letter home I get an ans. next mail. I get your ans. the 2nd mail. Do you get my letters that way? By the way, this is pretty near your birthday — you are 22 now if I remember rightly and almost a Dr. If I had been a Dr. at 22 I would have had my fortune made before this and would have nothing to do but spend it.

I hope you get lots of nice things on your birthday. There is not a thing in this town that I could send you, not even a native! Birthdays are very common to me now for I have seen about 3 or 4 a week for the last six weeks!

Now good bye and be _good_ & remember me to Miss Abbott and the little French Dr. Don't hurt yourself studying and be sure and write me all about the exams.

Dr. Cross, the cheeky one, is doing well making money and friends. I am going to pay him a visit shortly. I forgot to tell you what he said about you, He said "Well, do you know _she_ is a blamed nice little _thing_." "Gosh I made her blush like a fury." No wonder you call him "cheeky."

Sincerely your   Wm. C. Little

P.S. I mail you a photo of my house with Dr. Cross (cheeky) & myself standing in front. I tell you who we are for I am sure you would not know if I didn't!

(Rec. April 24, 1891
Ans. May 27, 1891)

Warracknabeal
March 20, 1891

My dear Grace,

I have just this moment discovered that the Frisco mail goes out tomorrow and I have only abt. one hr. to write you. I shall not be able to write home this mail.

It appears your prognosis is coming true about "letters being shorter and shorter and greater distance apart." I missed the last mail by being out in the country. I had to drive 30 miles, which took me all day and all night as it was a bad case. When I got back the mail had *gone.*

I am busy as ever, sometimes quite done out. I have had a lot of bad cases which have given me a good deal of anxiety. I have had 3 cases of Septicemia, with one death, and I religiously stick to autopsies. You have no idea how such cases trouble me.

I have been called in consultation several times lately. I have to meet a Dr. in consultation this afternoon.

I must not forget to tell you that we have a hospital here now and I am the Surgeon, for which I receive $500 a year.[45] I will only have to visit it once a day.

A new shire has been formed here so they will want a health officer at a salary of $200 a year, so I am now on the lookout for that. There is nothing like being ambitious. I love to keep getting higher and higher. I think you are like that also. I have been so busy I cannot get a day to visit my cousin Dr. Cross.

I hope you will be able to read this scrawl. I know if I don't write this time I will be forever in your black book. Now that you are a Dr. I know you will have a little more sympathy than before, as you will more fully realize how much his time is taken up.

I did not rec. a letter from you this mail, at the same time I can quite excuse you as I know every moment of your time was taken up with examination work. I shall anxiously await the results. However, I know the results without hearing them — "passed with honors."

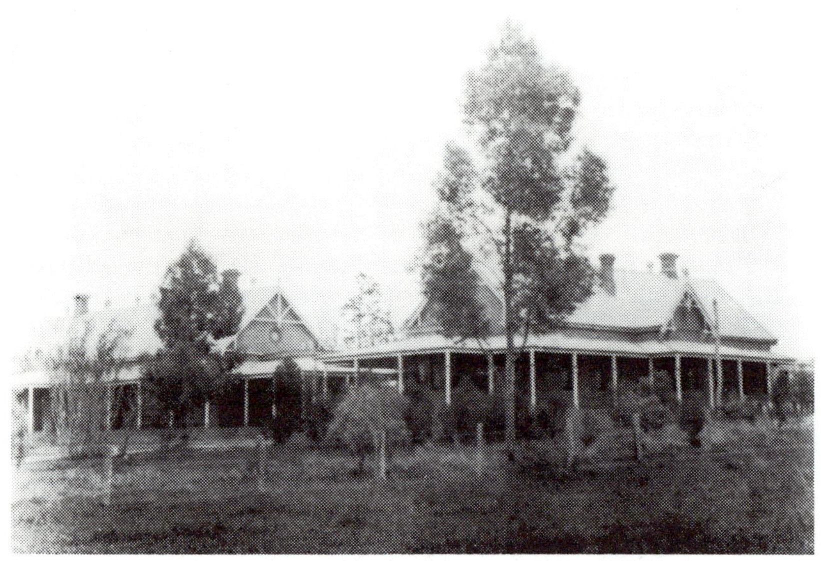

The Warracknabeal Hospital in the 1890s

To refer to your letter about our becoming strangers to each other, well, there is no necessity for that. I think we can be honest with each other and just say what we think. There is no doubt, let any two friends be separated for a long time — the fact that their time is fully occupied with business or professional duties must make in time a difference in intensity of friendship. Yet they remain friends [just] the same.

Our lives at present are running in different directions, but the Lord only know[s] but they meet somewhere.

Since I wrote you last, I have bought a property $2500 cash, so that I now live in a house of my own. I am beginning to feel quite important now. So will you when you get a house and a good practice. The latter is certainly the most pleasing.

I am slowly getting into Australian ways and habits — not the bad ones, as I had enough before I came here.

The hospital committee have advised that I go to Melbourne to buy surgical instruments and other necessaries for the hospital. I expect they will pay expenses. I shall be glad of a day or so's rest.

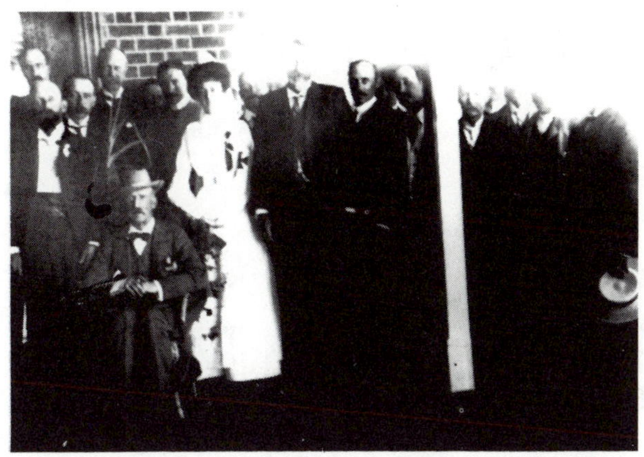

The opening of the Warracknabeal Hospital in 1891. Dr. Little is third from left

By this time you will have your mind fully made up about going to England. You will enjoy the trip so much. I just wish I could meet you there. I would ask the privilege of taking you to some of the operas and places of amusement.

Do you ever hear from Miss Demerest and Mrs. Walker and if so, what are they doing? I did not see a scratch of a pen from Canada this mail.

I was quite interested in the Canadian elections. I see by telegrams that J.A. Macdonald still remains premier.[46] He is a wonderful man. I remember him saying in 1886 that he would be premier after that election and that he would be premier after the 1891 election. Far-seeing old rascal. Still I admire him.

I have spent some time lately reading up hypnotism. I have tried it on a few subjects with slight results. I have put a patient to sleep, etc. I believe I could mesmerize you. What do you think?

You would make an excellent hypnotist, I am sure. Just try it on some of your poorer patients.

I have just ten minutes to finish and get to the post so I must say good bye and ask you to forgive my miserable letter. I shall try and improve in future.

After this I shall have to address you as Dr.

I am

Sincerely yours,
W.C. Little

(Rec. Edinburgh June 8, 91
Ans. Glasgow June 25, 91)

Warracknabeal
April 14, 1891

My dear Grace,

Here I am sitting comfortably in my dining room, a beautiful fire burning in the grate & the rain gently falling on the roof so that I have calmly sat down to write you, feeling that I will not be disturbed. Could I bring myself to believe that thousands of miles did not separate us, I could quite easily make this letter as our long chats used to be — what were they, a mixture or compound? — pretty much mixture, I think.

I must tell you before going farther that your letter of Feb. 27 came to hand earlier than you expected and it is the best letter I have had from you for 3 or 4 months. In fact it pleased me and made me feel better for — well, the effects have not worn off yet.

Life with me is just the same pretty much week after week — some get sick and get well, others get sick and die. Even these things become monotonous.

During the past month I have been called in consultation three times by 3 different Drs. and strange to say, two of them were placenta praevia cases.[47] I have heard I did myself credit — "Oh you conceit," I hear you say. Well, no, I do not feel conceited any more than any man should feel and that is just enough to carry me through life in a kind of a way.

I took notice of what you said about settling down in a small place like Warracknabeal. Well, you are right probably, but to emigrate to a city might be a mistake. I do feel this place so narrow outside my profession. I have no nice places to spend my evenings, and the society I do meet is very often dull and uninteresting. So far as my profession is concerned, this is a good place. I live well and am kept busy. In Melbourne there are many Drs. who do not make as much in one year as I make in a month. At present I could not settle down in a city and wait day after day, yr. after yr., for a few straggling patients to come to me. — It would be hell to me. I cannot live unless I am busy. It is essential to me, I would go to the devil if I were not kept busy.

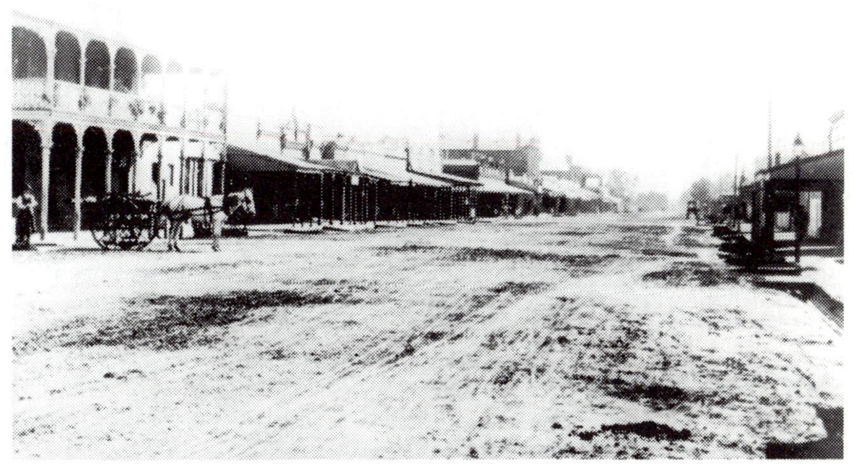

Warracknabeal circa 1894

I got hold of a German grammar a few weeks ago but, bah, I cannot study the stuff. I would like to be able to talk German as there are many here. My mouth cannot form the words, besides I have not a teacher. A lady offered to teach me, but I feared I would talk more English and bosh than German.

I must tell you my latest fad — Hypnotism or suggestive Therapeutics. I have been studying the above for about one month and have had three patients.

No. 1 — lady had headache for two days. I hypnotized her in two minutes that she could not open her eyes, do what she would. Headache cured in 3 minutes, not returned 13 hrs. afterwards.

No. 2 patient — ostitis and periostitis, great pain. I gave a dose quinine gram $\bar{v}$, which left bad taste in his mouth. I hypnotized him, made him believe the tongue tasted sweet — which he positively asserted, and removed for a time the ostitis pains.

No. 3 — boy — 9 years old with foreign body imbedded in cornea. I hypnotized him, had him asleep in two minutes and removed foreign body without pain. I stuck a pin in him ½ inch and he did not move. I could wake him up and make him go to sleep at will. I related the above to a Dr. lately from Ireland. He did not believe me. As no. 3 was to come to surgery last Saturday, I invited the Dr. to come and see for himself. The boy seemed happy and wide awake when he came in. I had him sit on a chair and told him he would have to go to sleep again. He said he would not. I said yes, you must and you will be sound asleep in 1½ minutes. In less than that time he was sound asleep. I lifted him up and placed him on a sofa, operated on his eye, stuck pin in him, waked him up, ordered him to go to sleep again, which he did almost instantly. The Dr. was very much surprised and, to say the least of it, looks on me as some supernatural being. The above is quite true. I have a half idea you will think I am telling fairy tales. No one was more surprised than myself when I hypnotized No. 1. Now I am sure I can hypnotize 6 out of every 10, or 4 at least. You notice I do not use the term mesmerism. Oh no, not after Allens.

You will hear more from me on this fascinating subject as I feel sure I can use it to good advantage in my practice. Children are very susceptible to hypnotism. After I get more proficient, I shall give you all the necessary information how to do it.

"Suggestive Therapeutics" by H. Bernheim, M.D., Professor in Faculty of Medicine, Nancy, is the best work on Hypnotism. I wish I had known how to hypnotize when at Allens. I would have had some fun. I could have had you singing beautiful songs to imaginary charmed audiences etc. etc., Miss Bennett selling books by the hundreds, Miss Demerest in love with all the world and wishing to live 100 yrs., Mrs. Fair to sleep soundly and not wander around at night — and as docile as a lamb. Old man Allen holding his wife in loving embrace. Then across the street I would have had some more fun. Oh, why was I so ignorant? & now an intruder comes to the door. He does not know how to pull the bell, he must be from the country.

Poor Sam has to get the horses and I have 11 miles to drive to see a sick child. No more tonight so good-bye and if you were here, I am sure you would wish me a pleasant trip.

April 15 — Child had pertussis[48] with slight congestion of right lung. I am feeling rather dull this evening being out late last night & busy today. This was baby day or vaccination day, any amount of squalling.

I am invited to a bazaar tomorrow afternoon to purchase some fancy things. I have not many fancy things; on the mantle is a marble clock worth

$25, 2 vases, 2 swans' eggs and an Emu's Egg. Several pipes, cigars and the Menagerie, Etc. etc.

By the way, I took 4 days' holidays last week and visited my cousin — the cheeky one. I read him the part of your letter which referred to him. He says he was cheeky and that you named him properly. The truth of the matter was he had been partying with some friends who considered a party without wine or something else stronger was a tame thing indeed. I suspected as much when you wrote me after his arrival. Well, Cross is doing well and much liked.

When you rec. this, you will be acting in the capacity of a nurse. You should make a good nurse — you have the gentle touch & how a gentle touch soothes a patient. A proper touch gives confidence. So you will have to wash the baby. Mind its eyes. I'll tell you of a roguish plan I had laid for you in Kingston but it did not come off. I tried to get a confinement case but did not succeed. If I had I was going to invite you and Mrs. Walker and *make* you wash the baby. Sorry it did not come off, aren't you?

You will look quite motherly with the little possum on your knee.

So you are going to Edinburgh and where not. If you go to France, go to the Nancy School of Medicine and learn hypnotism. You could do it quite well. Your eyes are just the right sort.

Thanks very much for the birthday card, it is quite nice. It is very easy to remember my birthday but yours is on no day at all — it is hard to remember it. Only 23 yrs. old and an M.D., Ch.M., M.C.P.S.O., B.A. — great heavens, if I had been as clever as you, today I would be worth $100,000 and could settle down in the city not caring whether patients came to me or not. Well, I had not the opportunity, so its no use crying over the past. My father has offered me a nice brick house if I will go home and settle in Toronto. It does not suit me, so I shall remain here until I am suited.

Patients are beginning to come to the new hospital, 5 in all now. I have also a private hospital where I send patients to. It pays me very well. I had three broken ribs, a broken arm and a broken leg to set last week after I came home. I removed quite a large cystic tumor today. I saved a woman from the fiendish grasp of a quack who was going to remove her breast — for cancer, when there was no cancer at all.

I played my big cousin, Dr. Cross — the one you haven't seen — three games of billiards for $2.50 a game and beat him. Isn't that good? It is only when I am taking holidays that I gamble a bit. I know it is wrong, but then I love to do wrong things sometimes for experience sake.

I have not had my photo taken yet, but will do so as soon as the photographer recovers from his present illness. I have just ordered a new suit of clothes in Melbourne so I shall wait until they come. I am getting a great coat for winter; it will be about one inch thick and down to my heels. I do not want to run any risk of getting congestion of the lungs.

It is acknowledged that I have the prettiest pair of horses in the town. They are lovely and wild.

I have just finished reading a book, "The World of Cant." I liked it very much. It exposes all the shams of religion and the motives which prompt the many to join themselves to churches etc. It is well worth reading, but quite likely you have already read it. I generally read myself to sleep every night, which is practically an auto-hypnotism.

You must have found it very dull at College with no lady friends with you, but that is all over now. It does seem such a short time since you started the study of medicine and now you have authority to heal the sick. Now, do you feel any taller or just the same? The feeling I had was "Thank God, exams are over and I can now begin to study." If I were you I would not give much attention to Surgical work, for you will get little of it to do. If you go to Edinburgh, it will pay you best to attend the children's hospital and the medical wards. I gave too much time to surgery. I get a good deal of it to do. I was called in consultation a short time ago to a supposed dislocation of the elbow which the Dr. could not reduce. It was a fracture of the upper third of the ulna. The time I spent on surgery has certainly given me a confidence which I find is very important.

Well, well, my monotonous life must roll on until next October at which time, if all goes well, I am going to visit South Australia. I believe it possesses many attractions in the way of scenery. I have found [it] so hard to tie myself down to steady work. Fancy nine months without a holiday. I never did so faithful work before. I certainly envy you your trip to England; but why be covetous since I have had my day and now I must settle down.

Let me see, in 1893 the Chicago Exposition is to take place, and that is the time when I left home that I purposed returning. That will be two more years yet. Oh, by that time you will be a professor in the Montreal Ladies Medical College, i.e., according to your chart. A professor, just fancy! I suppose you will scarcely deign to look upon an ordinary practitioner then. That is your doom if there ever is a ladies' College in Montreal. How do you like it — Dean of the Faculty?

Do you know since you told me I am not to think of you as you were at Allens, I feel lost. I only knew you as you were there and now I am to think of you as someone else. It is devilish hard, in fact, I cannot do it. I must either think of you as the same jolly, innocent girl or I, knowing what latent ability you have, place you quite beyond me, in which position I naturally feel strange. Supposing I tell you not to think of me as you knew me — think of me as a great big bald-headed crosseyed Dr., front teeth all out, except the eye teeth, which project over my lips a foot — think of me standing beside a patient's bed, the terror of me either producing sudden cure or quicker death, think of me ha! — ha! — ha! ha! You can't do it. Not much — you think of me as you knew me.

To be honest, I liked you very much as I knew you but if you are quite transformed, I might not like you a bit. Well, you will have a laugh over this and I have no doubt will quietly whisper to yourself, "likes or dislikes do not matter to me." Well mind, don't let the baby fall or you will hear from your sister.

Are you coming out to Australia & home by Frisco after doing the continent? It would be a grand trip and would give you at least a lease of 10 extra yrs.

When you go to Edinburgh give me your address as I want to buy or I want you to let me buy you a morning gown the same as the old one, wine color I think; you see I can't send things from here very well to Canada. I shall not forget, No. 6. Have you had the cast taken yet? I have the finger and the tooth yet, came across them the other day. I lost the pin you gave me and I cannot find it. It came out of my tie somehow.

I have just 15 minutes to get to the post office.

I am yours
the same as you knew me,
W.C. Little

Miss Grace Ritchie B.A., M.D., Ch.M.
Address I don't know where

Warracknabeal
June 11, 1891

My dear Grace,

I received your very welcome letter of April 2nd to hand in due time, also the paper with account of convocation in it. I was delighted to hear how nicely you got on with your exams. You got through without a hitch. Isn't it a relief to the mind to feel all you have to do is either to go into practice or better still, to more thoroughly fit yourself for life's work.

To simply write "I congratulate you" would not convey my feelings. I think you have done remarkably well & have accomplished a very great deal during your yet short life. I was pleased to notice that all spoke so nicely of you at convocation. The ladies in Arts did not forget you. I do hope they did not forget to put a few lovely roses in the wreath you were presented with. I know you are fond of roses, especially before a medical reunion. Well, you are fond of excitement and I fancy you had plenty of it the day you were knighted M.D., Ch.M. I do wish I could have been there. I can assure you had I been within 500 miles I would have been there. 15,000 miles! what a terrible distance & here I am writing you and not knowing what part of creation you are in. I cannot locate you. I have tried to see if my feelings would tell me but, alas, the distance is too great.

Well you are a big medical dr. now and I have no doubt will perform many wonderful cures and I suppose considering that I am *barred* from thinking of you as I *knew* you, I will have to write quite a professional letter. I don't believe I can do it as it makes me feel as if I had a big collar and a heavy harness on. Well, to tell you the truth, I do not feel that way in the least. The fact of the matter is your letter was so natural, so much like yourself as I knew you, that we are quite good friends again, providing you will forgive all the nasty things I wrote in my last letter, which by the way, you had not rec. when you wrote last.

Well, Grace, I wish I could be in the old country with you if it were only for a fortnight. I did like it so much. I like London. You will find there is a great deal to learn when you visit the large hospitals. Try & hear some of the big lights in the MD profession — Royal Sir Jas, and if in Edinburgh, Byron Bromwell, Granger Stewart and a host of others. When in France go

> **THE FIRST LADY GRADUATE**
>
> **In Medicine in Quebec Province Gets Her Diploma Yesterday.**
>
> ———
>
> **BISHOP'S CONVOCATION.**
>
> ———
>
> **Mr. Justice Tait Receives the Honorary Degree of D. C. L.—Addresses by the Chancellor of the College, the Dean of the Faculty and Others.**
>
> ———
>
> The annual convocation of the University of Bishop's college, held yesterday afternoon in the Synod hall, will be memorable in the annals of medicine in the province of Quebec, inasmuch as it witnessed the conferring of the degree of C.M., M.D. for the first time in this province upon a lady. The lady who has earned this proud distinction is Miss Octavio Grace Ritchie, who, along with others, was instrumental in getting the doors of at least one medical college in this province thrown open to ladies.

"Clever girl"

to Nancy where they carry on many interesting experiments in hypnotism. I noticed your valedictorian spoke of hypnotism as a therapeutic agent, etc.

In my last letter I told you I was devoting a good deal of time to the study of hypnotism. I have the very great satisfaction to tell you that I am now a hypnotist of no ordinary ability — I mean ability to hypnotize. I have now, in all, some 20 or 25 cases, [in] all of which I have observed beneficial results. To give you a history of them all would fill two letters, so I shall confine myself to a few.

One case I produced deep sleep and complete anaesthesia so that another Dr. curetted the uterus without the patient feeling anything. Another case I opened a felon[49] on finger, cutting right down to the bone; no feeling. Another case, extracted two teeth and opened abscess — no pain. Another case — insomnia cured by three visits, besides, a host of others for neuralgia, headaches, etc. I am treating a case which I think will turn out to be very interesting. Labourer, 33 yrs. old, married, suffering from epilepsy ever since 25 yrs. of age. Has been under some six Drs. He consulted me a little over a week ago. I recommended him to let me hypnotize him, since drugs had proved of no avail, to which he consented. He had been in the habit of having 3 & 4 fits during the week and sometimes 2 in one day. I had no difficulty hypnotizing him — had him completely under in two minutes. I was astonished to find I could induce a cataleptic condition, could make the arm, leg or all the body perfectly rigid. I could paralyse the arm, leg, eye, tongue and speech — any one at will. I then made him talk and had him repeat after me, "During the week I shall not have any fits; I shall be perfectly well and happy." This I had him repeat several times. I also told him to come and see me the following Monday at 5 p.m. On awaking he knew nothing of what I had said to him. He had a severe occipital headache, which never left him for ½ an hour at a time. This, I removed in two seconds. I sent him home and told him to come to see me when he felt he should. To my surprise he came to the surgery door precisely at 5 p.m., he had to quit work ½ an hour early to do so. I asked him why he came and at that particular hour. He said it occurred to him every day that he must see me on Monday evening. Results: he had no fits during the week, the headache did not return and he never felt happier in his life.

I hypnotized him a 2nd time and had him repeat the same words and to come and see me on Monday at 7:30 p.m. On awaking he knew nothing of what I had said to him.

He is quite an athlete, the second best wrestler in the town. I said to him, "I believe you are a good wrestler." He said, "Yes, I can throw any man in the town bar one." I said, "I will wager you £10 to £1 that I can throw you." He said I could not. I told him to get up and we would try, which he did. I paralysed every limb in his body and took him and laid him on his back on the floor, telling him at the same time he could not get up. He could not move hand or foot. He admitted I was too strong for him and gave me best.

I shall tell you more later on about this interesting patient and what control I have over the fits.

Altho I can hypnotize I do not understand what effect it produces on the brain. Why is it one can suggest to another and they cannot help being governed by that suggestion? It is a very strange thing and difficult to explain. Young and old are subject to it. The other day I amputated a child's tonsil, the child knew nothing about it until I wakened her to spit out the blood.

Now, Grace, do not think I am becoming a crank on this subject, & likely to degenerate into a quack, far from it. I am perfectly satisfied [that in] many cases, particularly when troubles are largely imaginary, hypnotism will prove very beneficial. On the other hand, what a power to have over human beings, a power which alike could be used for bad as well as good.

Why, I could send that man home with a suggestion to chastize his wife twice a day and he would do it. What a power for a barrister to possess. He could make a witness swear lies were truth and all sorts of things.

I am going to try and get a man who is addicted to drink and try and cure him. I can suggest that the whiskey is poison and tastes fearfully bitter, etc.

Life with me is pretty much of a sameness. I am kept busy now and again having a surgical operation to vary the programme. I have a big toe to amputate this week. The hospital is full of patients who take up a part of my time. I have all the babies in the district to vaccinate and the general health of the town to look after, so that I have not much spare time to myself. I think I am standing the work pretty well. I am weighing well, which is a fair indication.

The photographer was at my house the other day when I came in from my rounds. He took a photo of the horses, house, garden, etc. There were some patients waiting my return. I mail you one of the photos with this. My own photos will not be finished in time for this mail, but will be ready as soon as I get your Old Country address. If you have had any of your photos taken I would be so delighted to get one. I promise you I shall have it framed nicely and put in the nicest corner in the house. I am anxiously waiting to hear what kind of passage you had over the ocean, how sick you were. I believe you would be sick just for wishing that I would when I was crossing the Atlantic. Did you see any porpoises and if so, what did you think of your friends? You will have any amount of things to write about, seeing new things every day.

I think it is time to have a smoke now, especially as there are a few tempting cigars near by. You should see what a pretty little 3-legged smoking table I have. It is a present from a grateful patient. It is in the shape of a horse shoe with a place for cigars, pipes, matches & ashes.

I had a little surprise party a few nights ago; a gentleman and 4 ladies called on me about 9 p.m. I know they called just to see how an old bachelor lives. I had things quite cosy, treated them to coffee, cake, cigars if they wanted them and best of all a *Canadian pie,* a thing they had never seen before. They seemed to like it. The chaperone, a married woman, begged a piece to take home to her husband. We had a real enjoyable hour. I had a visit from my cousin, Dr. Cross, sr. and the manager of the National Bank. They had dinner with me on Monday. As luck would have it another grateful patient had on Saturday previous made a present of two fine fat wild ducks. My cousin is a jolly fine fellow and a good man in his profession.

I really like practice in this country. You would be surprised the great difference between practice here and in Canada. Patients think nothing of coming into the town and staying 3 or 4 days to be treated, & often for trivial ailments. A Dr. is much more respected here than at home. It is noticeable on the street, for when I am driving along even the labouring class will lift their hats. Altho there is not much in it, yet I cannot help feeling the honor.

I was consulted by a Member of Parliament a few weeks ago. He came back to tell me he was cured and he seemed downright thankful.

My professional life I enjoy very much. Oh, I was consulted by letter by a patient 500 miles from here — in Adelaide. This patient had heard somehow of another patient who had suffered from the same complaint and I had cured. I received a 2nd letter yesterday to say there was much improvement. You would never hear of a patient at home leaving the city Drs. to consult a country Dr. These are some of the brightnesses I have in life. Yet socially I do not feel satisfied. I don't think I have improved a bit since you saw me last. This is sad, isn't it? The fact of the matter is, I have no one to correct me or call my attention to little improvements which might be made. I could do any outlandish thing and it would at once be excused by "Oh, that's American."

It is now fast approaching 1 a.m. and as the mellowing, soothing and hypnotic effects of the *good* cigar are working on me, my mind feels like standing still for awhile, which if I allow it to do, sleep will be the result.

Did you ever notice that after midnight your mind turns to things stern and oft-times sad? I think if I had to preach a sermon I would make it all up after midnight. It would be full of very original ideas about life and mortality and what not, that the vast audience would yawn off to sleep.

Poor Sir John A. Macdonald has gone the way of all flesh. He was a wonderful statesman, the cleverest man in Canada. He was clever inasmuch that he knew men and their ways so thoroughly that it made him a master leader.

Sarah Bernhardt is creating a sensation out here. The people of Melbourne are fascinated with her. She is even a greater success in her life than John A. She simply holds the audience in raptures. I suppose you had the pleasure of seeing her in Montreal.

My brother, who is now in Sydney, will have the honor of seeing her act. I have not seen my brother for six months. He is coming up in October when he, Dr. Cross and myself are going to Adelaide for a few weeks' holiday.

I am sorry you did not get my letter at the time you expected. I don't think you ever expected a letter from me as much as I did one from you one time and I did not get it. When I really expect a letter and don't get it, it makes me simply mad. It may have missed the mail, if so, it was not my fault for it was mailed in plenty of time. This letter will reach you as fast as if it went by the canal. Don't forget to tell me about anything new in surgery or medicine you may learn while sojourning in Europe. I simply envy you your trip and experience, yet at the same time your education will not be anything like complete unless you visit the large hospitals of Australia.

I shall anxiously await your address. You know I won't know whether you are drowned or not until I get it. Of course you could swim ashore. Porpoises do not as a rule die of drowning.

Now good bye and I hope you will have a pleasant and profitable sojourn in foreign lands. Good night.

I remain your
sincere friend
Wm. C. Little

— Now don't read this page until you have read all the others as I missed it somehow or other. Glad to hear your sister made a good recovery. Sorry the little one chipped through the shell a month too soon — better luck next time. You have never told me anything about Mrs. Savage this long time. You see I have not forgotten her yet. Do you know she possesses a peculiar wit — which I have not met before. You see when anything out of the ordinary strikes me I don't forget it.

I suppose Miss Abbott will be mourning your departure. Tell her I have not forgotten her when you write. I think that is quite as good as sending love, especially if you're not sure about it.

My worldly goods are gradually increasing. I have a Swan, two ducks, some hens and I believe chickens expected soon.

P.S. This letter is pretty long & I fear so badly written you'll hardly be able to read it.

Did Miss Bennett recover from her illness?

This is a pepper tree leaf.

(Rec. August 21, 1891, London
Wrote August 19, before rec. this.)

Warracknabeal
July 9, 1891

My dear Grace,

I am here cooped up in my dining room, a beautiful fire on, which makes the dreary night a little pleasant. I am invited out for the evening to some parlour musical affair with probably a game of cards, a waltz and so on to make up the evening. Well, like a certain night in Kingston, I think I prefer to remain at home and spend the evening with you. Now, don't you think that is very good of me? To spend an evening with you so far away seems almost impossible, yet I believe there is nothing impossible to the imagination. So now I will give you the comfortable rocking chair by the fire to listen while I tell you all my tales of woe and otherwise.

Your letter from Edinburgh dated May 26 came to hand last Friday night. Your letter was a surprise to me. It just seemed to come in, in the right place. I was thinking of the Frisco Mail, so your letter stole in on me unawares. I was delighted to rec. it, in fact it made me feel quite a new man, you seemed so bright and so natural. You know when you rec. something you like and did not expect it just then and you get it, well, that's how I felt. The fun of it was I had a Billiard tournament match to play that night in a private house and I had to play one of the Champions with a start of 70 points ahead of my opponent. He had said he would have no difficulty in beating me. I just felt in the right humor and in a positive self-confidence feeling, which never left me and which had a depressing effect on my opponent. I never played a better game. Every shot was as careful and as well calculated as possible. The result was he never caught me. All present were delighted with the game I played. Alas, a dark cloud appeared in the person of a messenger for me to go 15 miles in the country to see a sick child. I was out all night & did not get home the next day until 11 a.m.

July is the dreary month of the yr. in Australia. There is not even a ray of beauty in it. This is the very heart of winter — it should not be called winter for it lacks the beautiful snow and the frost. The ground is never frozen, it is simply a sodden old rug. The atmosphere is chilly and damp, the roads are mud and slush, the trees, which shed their bark instead of their leaves, are dripping with water instead of being beautifully iced over like the Canadian forests. If this letter has any complaining in it, do for heaven's sake blame this miserable month for it and not me. Flat country makes a person feel flat; sodden country sodden. Poor Australians, I pity the poor swag men. They tramp from one part of the country to another looking for work. They carry their own bed, which consists of a piece of sail cloth and a blanket. The poor devils have to sleep outside under a gum tree these dreary nights. Is it any wonder when they get a little money that they drink it all? It is the only pleasure they ever have and it is a good way to forget their troubles.

You are a porpoise in truth or you would have been sea-sick. There is no doubt about it, you had a touch of it. Lovely feeling, isn't it? I believe that a big bag full of things you got kept you from being sea-sick. I can imagine without the slightest difficulty how you would examine the contents of that bag. You had them all out on yours or your mother's cabin bunk, just the way you used to get all your treasures spread out around you at the drum at 40 Stewart St. I am sure you felt as if you were only 15 years old and probably even younger than that. You forgot the B.A., M.D., Ch.M. with the coming addition of L.R.C.S.E., L.R.C.P.E. Fancy all those letters looking over a bag full of trinkets. I am blamed if I know what Glycerin and rose water is used for. You made me curious by saying you shouldn't mention them to me. What are they for anyway?[50]

There goes jingle at the bell, blame the luck — Well, it was an old Irish woman, a farmer's wife, very well to do. Their cattle got into a big field of grass and their stomachs are swelling up very large, so she wanted to know if I could give her something to let the wind out of them. Great United States, this is fun. I gave her the largest trocar I have and told her or showed her how to stick it in and the wind would come whistling out. She was so serious I dare not laugh at her. I told her if she could not get the wind out of them quick enough with the trocar to stick a knife into them. I do hope she manages to save the lives of the poor dumb animals.

I have just rec. papers from Sydney concerning the horse races. There is a big sweep, a kind of a lottery. I shall take two tickets in it — one for you and one for myself. You see we stand a chance of winning from £10,000 to £100. Now, if I win the £10,000 I am to give you ½ and if you win you are to give me half. I shall have your ticket labelled "Porpoise, Warracknabeal" so if you see anything of it in the papers you will know who it means. The tickets are only 10/- each.

This is an awful country for horse racing, betting, gambling and drinking. As one writer has put it, birds without song, flowers without smell, and women without ——. Well, I believe I have forgotten one thing, I know it is not flattering to the women, but I do not believe it a bit.

I was nearly forgetting that you are sitting in the chair by the fire. I must stir it up a bit or you might catch cold & it is so fearfully wet outside I am afraid you will have to stay all night as I have left my umbrella I don't know where.

So you are in Edinburgh now, the fine old city. Don't you think Montreal compares very favourably with it? Do you know I have come to the conclusion that there are few prettier places than Montreal, of course barring Lachute. How do you like the Cowgate, the Canongate and the Meadows? What do you think of the Infirmary?

Dear me, I have just stopped for a while to have a smoke and there goes the bell — I have to go to the country & there is no knowing when I shall get back. I must after this letter begin my letters 3 or 4 days before the mail goes out to ensure that they will be finished. If I get back before 3 in the morning I shall finish this, so good night and I am sorry I cannot finish my evening with you.

I have just returned from the country cold as ice. Placenta Praevia case; woman nearly died. I delivered child in 5 minutes. Charged $75 for case.

Could you not forward me an Old Country address so if I miss the Frisco mail I could send by P. & O.

3 minutes to mail time.

Good-bye
Sincerely your
W.C. Little

(Rec.
Ans.)

Warracknabeal
August 7, 1891

My dear Grace,

I intended to begin this letter two days ago in order to insure its completion, as the last one I sent you was about ½ finished.

Your letter of June 26 came to hand in good time, reached me about the time the American mail came in. Yes, you are farther from me now than you were in Montreal. So you think you will not go home by Australia. It is a great mistake as you may never have a better chance of seeing the world or going around it at least. When you settle down to the responsibility of a practice, there is very little time for holidays. You have to work hard to get a practice together and when you do succeed, you have to exert yourself equally as much in order to keep it together. I never knew what tied down meant until I came here. As time goes on I get entangled in business & professional duties which require my time and attention and so time flies, and life rolls on at an unusual fast pace. Since writing you last I have been doing some investing in property. I have bought 1280 acres of land for which I was able to pay cash. I am hoping to double my money on it. I am about buying 640 acres more so that when I get that, I shall be quite a landed proprietor. I am on the look out for bargains, you know that is my weakness. I would even sell the bones of the dead at a profit. I hope you will also make a profit out of them. I am scarce of bones now so I had my groom go and dig up 4 black fellows' graves, but alas, they had cremated the bodies and the bones were all spoiled. I don't know that I ever got the better of you in a bargain unless it was on the Napanee trip when you had to pay your own expenses.

I believe I shall always be compelled to laugh over that trip and I am sure you will also feel the same. Fancy when you are a great grandmother relating that experience to your grandchildren.

When I wrote you last I was called to the country some 23 miles to a placenta praevia case. The patient had a very narrow escape. Had I been ½ an hour later she would have gone to heaven. Poor woman. She is now suffering from phlegmasia alba dolens.[51] Oh yes, I get such cases here. I am very busy now working night and day. I have been up four nights in succession attending confinements. Two of the cases were forceps cases and one post partum. Now I have something to tell you about hypnotism. I hypnotized a patient in labor and she told me that she scarcely felt any pain. I suggested to her that she would not cry out and strange to say, she never complained a bit, even when the head was being born. She was very nervous and said she would die if she did not get $CHCl_3$.[52] I called on her a week before & hypnotized her in order to be sure of my ground when labor did come on.

I notice your advice and will act accordingly; I always operate in presence of some other person. Do you suppose I could make a girl fall in love with me by suggestion? What a funny idea. Will you let me try it when next I see you? Oh, the man with the fits is getting better fast, hasn't had a fit for a long time. His memory has improved and I can make him sleep every night from 10 to 6, a thing he hasn't done for years. I could make this man do anything I like. I offered him 10 sovereigns one night if he would lift them off my hand, at the same time suggesting that he would not be able to touch them. He could not take one of them. I showed this case to a Dr. from Tasmania and he was surprised I could cause complete paralysis of any groups of muscles and anaesthesia at will. I also showed this Dr. a case of Gastric Catarrh I had in the hospital who would not retain any food in the stomach and yet when hypnotized, she would keep a cupful of milk down for hours. The Dr. said he would give £1000 to be able to do it.

I do not think you will like Glasgow very well as it is a very dirty place. I spent about a week in it. McEwan is a good man on hernias and knock-knee operations. He is very original and gruff in his manner. He is inclined to be a bit rough on other Drs. at times, e.g. "Only a fool would do that" when just as clever a man as himself had done it. There is considerable rivalry between Glasgow and Edinburgh. I believe Glasgow is a good school. There is a fine university there. I have been through it: — the Museum, Cathedral and *Wax works* — by all means go to the latter.

I think you will find the teaching much more thorough in the Old Country than at home. I do wish I were where I could attend a post-graduate class for a couple of weeks each year. It would be so refreshing.

By the way, I had a lady call today to know if I would give lectures on ambulance work if a class were got up. Of course I did not refuse. If it ever comes to anything, I shall let you know. I would give the lectures at the hospital where there would be patients to practise on. I have 10 patients in the hospital now. I am going to do some skin transplantations some of these days.

I rec. a nice present a few days ago from the Methodist Minister's wife — a small table cover and a thing to hang on the wall for matches and pipes. How considerate of her to put a place in for pipes. Some person unknown as yet sent me a nice pair of shoes. I am puzzled to know from whom they came. I bought a square for my bedroom — a carpet which here is called a square. I am getting things quite cosy now and will soon have a home comfortable enough for a woman to live in, but where she has to come from remains a mystery.

So Joseph Bell made a mash on you by calling you *My dear child.* Let me see, did I not call you *my dear child* or *woman* one time and you took me to task quite severely for it, so that ever since I have not made bold enough to call you anything but *my dear Grace,* or *possum,* or *porpoise?* Joseph Bell is a very fine man, he was my examiner at the Infirmary and also at my oral. I amused him very much with what I am sure he thought were crude answers. He asked me what I would do in certain cases. I told him it altogether depended on what means I had at hand and then gave him two answers. When I signed my name, he put his hand on my shoulders and gave me his blessing.

I want you to tell me anything new or wonderful in the medical and surgical world that you may come across. I can recommend you a good work if you do not already possess it. Dr. Castor's *"Physical Diagnosis."* Get the lastest edition of it. Diagnosis is quite simple in the majority of cases but there are the many cases extremely difficult. I treated a patient in the hospital and cured her and yet I never made out what she was suffering from. I had a patient die not long ago and I had some difficulty inventing a death certificate. There are constitutional diseases which partake of the nature of ½ dozen diseases and yet it is none of them.

You will feel very much annoyed and humiliated when you are brought face to face with a serious illness and yet you cannot honestly say what is the matter. In very many cases I recognize what is the matter the minute I see the patient. I had a case six months ago in which I diagnosed abscess of the lung and yet I was partially right and a bit wrong. The truth was he had an hydatid cyst in the lung. The hydatid died, which changed to an abscess which burst and to the friends proved what a clever Dr. I was. Yet I was wrong and I should have recognized it at once and tapped as it would have saved him months of illness. Drs. often get credit for ignorance and censure for remarkable skill.

I do all in my power to find out what is really the matter with every patient. I have a very peculiar case at present with all the symptoms of

Locomotor Ataxia [53] less all the painful ones. I have diagnosed it Friedreich's disease. [54] I am not certain about it as I have never seen a case. I am going to send him to the best man on nervous diseases in Melbourne to get his opinion.

So you liked Byron Bromwell. I am glad for I think a great deal of him. I am so sorry you did not hear him at the out-patient clinic. He uses beautiful language and goes fully into all the details of the case.

I fancy when you are in practice you will often think of the Glasgow Dr. whose treatment is nil. You will find as I have done that Hilton's method of *rest* will often give you better results than medicines. Fully ⅓ of the patients I treat in the hospital are simply given a placebo and rest — the recoveries are satisfactory and the patients go out to laud the Dr. to the skies for curing them with nothing. Homeopathy is just as good as any other treatment in such cases. If you can get your hands on Hilton's book on "Rest and Pain," just read it carefully and you will be pleased with it.

Anything new in medical literature which is really valuable that you come across in your travels be good enough to let me know about it. I take the Annual of Universal Medical Sciences which is published in Philadelphia each year and contains the latest in medicine for the year. I do not hear much of Koch now. I am treating two cases of phthisis with Guaiacol [55] and it is giving most happy results. I am treating my anaemic patients with an albuminoid preparation of iron called Ferri Maleschi. So far it is very satisfactory. I must now stop for a while and go and see a case of Peritonitis.

I was nearly forgetting to tell you, I had such a strange dream the other night in which I saw you as distinctly as if you had been in reality. I also saw my sisters and a host of other people. To my great disappointment I did not get a word with you for when we were just a few feet from each other the pleasure and excitement wakened me up. I was as much annoyed as when I landed in Montreal and heard you had left the city. In the dream you did not look any older and you looked as full of mischief as ever — just the same as you did the night you got the better of the Chinaman 5 cts. I must say it is not at all flattering to you.

The best way for you to get your letters is to have them sent to your bank and they will be forwarded to any part you may go to.

It must be very nice for you to have your mother with you, at the same time it will be dull for her when you are out.

Do you ever hear from Miss Bennett and Dr. Demerest now? I have never written to Gilles or Jack Robertson since I came out here.

Dr. Cross wished to be remembered to the porpoise when I wrote. He often laughs over the yarns he told you.

If you never see Australia until you get a $50,000 practice, you would not be able to see it if you did come, for your eye sight would be gone. I should not discourage you for you might at any rate do ⅓ of it, not in Montreal though.

Now good-bye and be good as you always are and remember if I do not write you the nicest of letters I often think of you as the nicest of girls and some day we may meet in Lachute and run a race to the mill dam. It is now 11:30 p.m. & I must write a letter home to my mother. She wrote me such a nice long letter last mail. Just fancy, she prays for me every night. How good of her.

Your sincere friend,
W.C. Little

Post-script: I have had a splendid night's rest and I got up early, have seen all my patients and find I have ½ hr. now before the mail closes. It's such a beautiful day, I feel happy and glad I am alive. My garden is beginning to look pretty, I have an orange tree in it, a leaf of which I enclose. For the next two months the climate here is all any person could wish for. My holiday time will soon be at hand and with what delight I shall throw off the harness and all restraint and be myself once more, free from care and anxiety. These are times we all look forward to with pleasure. I think a man cannot enjoy a holiday half unless he has been hard worked.

I want you to give me your banking address for when I am taking holidays I might run across something you would like.

Once more good bye and may all good angels guard you in your wanderings.

Sincerely your,
W.C.L.

Warracknabeal
September 4, 1891

My dear Grace,

I see by the paper the Frisco mail goes out tomorrow so I have just three hours before mail closes.

I received yours of July 21st about a week ago. Do you know it takes longer for a letter to reach me from Glasgow than from Montreal. I am glad to hear you are getting on so nicely, notwithstanding the disappointment you have met with. So you have met some Victorians and cheeky at that. I believe all colonials are cheeky — you remember Cross! The Australian is rather cheeky or self-assertive. I think I have met the gentleman you referred to. I fancy he was with a party of us when we went to see the Forth bridge. Ask him if he were with a party in which Tom Robertson of Australia was one of the members, to see the Forth bridge about 15 months ago.

So Fergie married Miss Herd or Miss H. condescended to have him. May God bless them but if I had been Fergie, I would have found out a means of transplanting my affections elsewhere. Really, there is no understanding Love, it masters all other feelings and transforms the most consummate flirt into constancy.

I have a sore finger so I have to hold the pen between the index and middle fingers. This is my old way of writing and I believe it is better than any other way.

I would like to hear McEwan grinding you. He is a rough diamond and still you cannot help admiring him. Even a brute of a man is often more respected than the *very* nice *man*. Well, Grace, I am tired out. I work very hard. I have been busy night and day for the past two months. Altho there are two other Drs. here — one more than when I came here, yet I get anything of importance there is to do. If patients do not get well under the other Drs., they come to me to learn what I think. I have had a run of accidents lately, fractures, dislocations and sprains. I had a dislocation of the knee joint on Sunday night. I have a bad case of aneurysm of the artery of the aorta. I made a most happy hit three days ago. A patient was brought some 70 miles to consult me — young woman age 21. After thoroughly examining her, I diagnosed Hydatids of the right lung. I gave her a dose of quinine as her temp. was 103, after which I extracted a molar tooth, while extracting the tooth she gave 3 or 4 screams. The tooth came out all right. I sent her away with instructions to come back in a week and I would operate on her chest and remove the Hydatids. ½ an hour after leaving the surgery she was brought back to me with about a pint of hydatids in a cloth which she had coughed up. I think the screaming burst the sack. She will get completely well now. I will get no end of credit for this case as she had been under 3 other Drs. and they said she would not live long. You should have seen the joy that lit her face when I told her she had Hydatids and that I would take them out. The beauty of it was I had not long to wait to prove my diagnosis correct.

Oh, joyful news, I have found the lost *pin* — for heavens sake tell your sister I have found it, do not let her think it passed into careless hands, but that it is very much prized. If her feelings are very much hurt over your parting with it, tell her I shall not forget her the first time I go back to Canada and will try and find something Australian that will be nice and will make up for your want of appreciation. I suppose your sister would call me cheeky if you were to tell her that. Now you had better say this, "The lost pin is found and I would not have given it to *Billy* only that I thought so much of it myself." (Myself means *yourself*)!

I had my portrait taken by the local artist — I mail you one which I think will reach you. You will notice I am a bit fleshier than when the Menagerie was taken. I look a bit older and more sedate, I think. You will see by it I am not baldheaded yet. You know I expect to be baldheaded some day as my father is. Still, I may take after my mother in that respect.

My holiday time is fast approaching. I am arranging with a Dr. to take my practice next month.

My brother will be with me in a few days. I have not seen him for 11 months, so you see we see very little of each other.

So you are going to France. Don't forget the Hypnotic hospitals. I want you to tell me all about their methods of treatment and the cases that give the best results.

Life with me is pretty much of a sameness, work, work, nearly all the time. When I do try to have a few hours of recreation my groom comes to tell me someone is anxious to see me. I have only had 3 Sundays to myself since I came here. Some Sundays I am busy from morning to night. I have nothing to mark the time, it is one continuous whole. A week ago last Sunday I drove 65 miles. Some day when I get rich I shall settle down to a much easier life. I am often asked why I do not get married. I tell them that the woman I would think enough of to marry would be too good for a Drs.

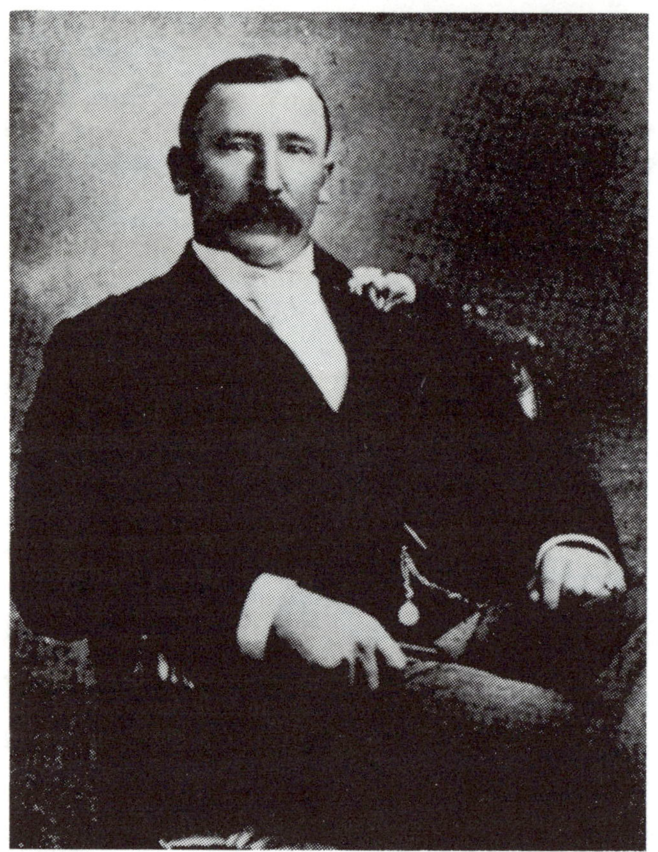

*"I had my portrait taken. . . . You will notice I am a bit fleshier. . . . I look a bit
older and more sedate, I think"*

wife and I would not like to take more than I could give. I am seldom at
home and when at home my time is thoroughly taken up.

In your travels try and find a cure for Varicose Veins other than
ligature, blistering, stocking bandage, injections and rubber bandage. If I
could get a positive and radical cure for varicose veins I could make a fortune.

If you come across anything new and good in the treatment of phthisis
I shall be glad to know of it. I am using Guaiacol and Cantharidate of Potash
with very satisfactory results.

When I can put my hands on the book you mentioned I shall read it. The Gods of this country are Drink, Gambling, and Making Money. It is about as hot a place for the above as can be found anywhere.

This letter is going to be a page short but the photo will make up as it will let you see I am well, etc. How I wish I could take my month's holiday in London. Wouldn't I enjoy myself! I do envy you the nice time you are having. This is a new kind of paper this time.

Now good bye, Grace, and may you always meet with kind hearts and kind friends and some day reach your ideal of $50,000.

Sincerely yours as ever
Wm. C. Little

(Rec. Vienna Dec. 15th '91
Ans. Feb. 8 & 26, 1892)

Warracknabeal
Oct. 29, 91

My dear Grace,

Your letter of Aug. 19th reached me a short time ago, the delay being I was away from home enjoying holidays. I was delighted to see your letter but when I came to answer it I find it is so long since I have written you that I hardly know where to begin. It might be just as well to begin by complaining, trusting that as I reach the end, I may develop a better frame of mind. In my last letter I told you how delighted I was that holiday time was coming. I have had my holidays but just 3 weeks shorter than I had anticipated. I rec. letters & telegrams to come back so often during the last week that I had to pack up and come home. The Dr. I got as Locum Tenens was so consummate lazy that he would not go out at night, the result was my patients went to the other Drs. My practice under his care fell off from 15-25 patients a day to 4-6. The lazy mope lost me $400 in three weeks. This Locum Tenens had great credentials from Edinburgh — had been house surgeon in a hospital in Liverpool, etc. and yet he and the other Drs. here could not recognize the urgent necessity of amputating an arm that had the principal arteries and nerves of the forearm completely destroyed. I found the arm and the patient in a terrible condition. I took the arm off at once and now the patient is recovering nicely from the septic condition I found him in. This is the first arm on the living subject that I have taken off. I came home at a most opportune time as the arm case has placed me complete master of the situation here. In one week I pulled my practice up from the 4-6 a day to 35 patients in one day, three of which I had to drive 30 miles in all to see. What a pleasing and stimulating effect it has to have the confidence of the people. Everything is right that I do. Nothing of the slightest seriousness is done by the other Drs. without having my approval. No, don't think I am blowing my own horn, I am just giving you my experience. I work hard, read the latest in medicine and surgery, which knowledge I put into practice as soon as possible so that it may become part of my implements of warfare.

I was worked very hard for 4 mos. before I took holidays and now I am worked harder than ever.

Now I must tell you a little about my holidays. I went to Adelaide in South Australia this time. I had called at Adelaide for an hour on my way out — so I knew very little about the place. I am delighted with Adelaide. It is a lovely city, so nicely laid out. No matter what direction you travel, you will find lovely little parks and groves and fountains. The Botanical Gardens are right in the centre of the city. So beautiful are they, I cannot describe them so if you ever want to know how lovely they are, you will have to come and see them.

I stayed at the best hotel, I believe the best in Australia, where everything is kept in the most perfect order. The proprietor and I got to be great friends; he took me out for drives and had me dine at his special table. I felt so well while there that I gained 10 lbs. in weight. I am quite proud of my appearance now. I am a good deal stouter than you ever saw me. I had a letter of introduction to the Mayor of the city. He was very friendly and nice. He called at the hotel one day and took me to dinner at parliament house, where I met the premier and some Sirs, etc., M.P.'s, and best of all, a good dinner.

My brother was in Adelaide with me and as he was very well acquainted I was never at a loss how to spend the time. It was three days before I could shake off the evil effects of overwork. One morning I wakened up and I started to whistle. I knew then I was right; I felt as if some terrible load was taken off me. My mind seemed so bright — I felt that life was a good thing and I was glad I was alive to be glad. I went to horse races, theatres, plays, American cowboys, review of the squadron, Roza Roza sports, played billiards, read novels and took a bath every morning. You will see my time was fully occupied and as nearly diametrically opposite to everyday routine of life as I possibly could devise. But the fates, the lazy Dr., the professional mope who wanted to get money without working for it, prevented me from taking a 3 days' sea voyage. I was wild about it. I am wild yet when I think of it. I do not like disappointments or [to be] crossed in my plans — there I go on the grumbling streak again, grumble, grumble and it does no good. Please excuse me, I should be all smiles and happiness while writing to you but then writing is such a prosy thing at best. I would rather talk to you for 2 hours than write the best possible letter my poor brain could imagine. I wonder if I can't hypnotize you and suggest that the only safe way to return to Canada is by way of Australia. I suppose I would have to hypnotize your mother also.

So you met Jack Shannon in London. He should have a good knowledge of his profession by this time. I believe Jack will do well. He has a nice address and good appearance, all of which should tell with the ladies. All a Dr. has to do is get the ladies, and the poor men must follow.

There goes the bell. I could swear, only I am learning to quit the use of bad words. It is a call to the country but as I know the patient's peculiar disposition, I sent out medicines with the promise to go in the morning. If you were here I would let you go if you liked for you would get $25 for the trip and you would be back in 2½ hours. I made $65 last Sunday in 5 hours. I charged $200 for amputating the arm and attendance. You can see it would never do for me to go back to Canada to practise medicine, I would charge too much.

So your mother thinks you write me too often and you ask me what I think of it. Well, I don't think you write too often. She is quite mistaken. She must think you are writing sometimes when you are not. No Grace, I am always delighted to hear from you. I am much interested in your welfare and nothing in the world pleases me better than to hear you are in good health, getting along well and showing a wee bit of interest in how I am getting on. To prove how glad I am to hear from you and a thousand times more to see you, I dreamt two different nights about you. The first, I thought my sisters and I were camping at some watering place. There were about 200 tents. One bright morning I was informed a new tent had been pitched and it was yours. I hastened away at once to find it.

While looking for it I suddenly met you and just as we were about to shake hands I started from my sleep.

The second time I met you I was in Adelaide and dreamt I was passing a university when curiosity prompted me to look in and I saw you writing in the far corner. You looked up and said, not "Billy," but "*Wm.*, come here." I walked in, sat down beside you, had scarcely spoken a dozen words when I wakened. You were as real as if I met you personally. The voice was as distinct and natural as possible. The pleasure was so great it wakened me and you know I am a good sleeper.

When I was in Adelaide I was looking around for something I thought you might like and the only thing I could find was a beautiful opossum robe. It will be nice to put over the back of a rocking chair, on the bed, or on the floor at the side of the bed or to use in driving. The first opportunity I have of sending it you shall get it in Montreal.

I saw some kangaroos when I was away. Saw one with a little one in her pouch. My next holiday is to Tasmania where I purpose going next

April if alive. I am going to take two holidays in the year. There is no sense in me killing myself. Life is too short for a man to make a slave of himself.

I have not the slightest idea where in the world this letter will find you.

Oh, I was nearly forgetting to tell you my friend, Shuttleworth, is married to a Guelph young lady — I rec. an invitation to the wedding but of course could not be present.

I notice what you say about rec. a proposal. I must say the young man was premature or he would have been surer of his ground before venturing. I admire his admiration so will not think too hardly of him.

Another poor sinner wants me. I shall finish this tomorrow morning. Good night.

Oct. 30

Dear Grace,

I got up early in order to get my work done so I could finish the letter and I cannot do it. I have two calls to the country which will occupy my time until past mail time.

I have some beautiful roses in my garden. I wish I could send you some. They are far prettier than those you got from Montreal.

Goodbye and remember I am always delighted to hear from you.

I remain your
Sincere friend,
Wm. C. Little

[There is a sixteen-and-a-half-month gap between this and the next letter.]

Launceston, Tasmania
March 15, 1893

My dear Grace,

You will see by the above that I am not at home. Delightful holidays, I am having them once more and all too short as they are, I shall spend the greater part of them on this little island. The dreams of my youth are being fulfilled in almost every particular. I remember when a boy at School studying the geography of Van Dieman's Land and how I thought when I became a man I would go and see it and its exiles. I became so worn out with practice, I could not take any interest, only forced interest in my work, so I wired away for another Dr. to relieve me. I was feeling quite down-hearted and not a bit myself until I came over here. The sea voyage simply pulled me together and now I am my old self again.

Not having any acquaintances here and not wishing to travel alone, I persuaded my brother to come with me, I to pay all expenses. Aren't you sorry you are not here? I have not tried what it is like to travel on other people's expenses but I fancy it must be lovely.

On Saturday last I paid a visit to the Flemington race course in Melbourne and saw one of the great events of the year. I made a little money backing horses — not enough to pay travelling expenses. A friend of mine made £2500.

The ruination of the Colonies is horse racing and betting. It is simply demoralizing the youth of this country — not a small part of the youth but 8/10 of them. Australia is simply a gambling hell. You hear nothing else from morning until night both in the parlor and on the street. I am afraid I am in the blues and may some day refute this bad opinion of Australians. I hope I shall be able to do so.

I have not had a letter from you for two months. I suppose you are very busy. I know if you are not busy, you will be some day. I think you have a nice manner for a lady Dr. and will succeed better than any of the "Menagerie."

If you are not busy you had better come out to Australia where I can get you plenty of work, without having to wait for it. How would you like a partnership basis? Just fancy, "Drs. Ritchie and Little, etc. may be consulted — hrs. 9-11 and 2-4." That would look all right. Well, let us get down to figures re partnership. I shall pay you $1000 first year, $1500 2nd year and $2000 3rd year. Don't you think me liberal? I think it is always nice to have a good offer ahead of you, it acts as a barrier to keep the wolf from the door and then you can say I have been offered so and so. Well, I suppose there would be little use trying to induce you to leave Montreal. I know you have good prospects there and I am sure you will do well. I have such faith in you, in fact more so than in any other *woman* living. Don't object to "woman" like you did once when I said 'My dear woman.'

Some day I shall drop in to your surgery quite unknown to you. When I do go home I shall not let any one know.

By the way, my cousin, Dr. Cross, is going home next month. He will be in Montreal likely. I shall give him your address and ask him to call on you. He is a fine fellow, a little outspoken but a real good man. He has plenty of money, about $100,000, so can afford to travel about whenever he likes.

That reminds me, I have a nice opossum robe for you & I shall get him to take it with him and he can send it from Toronto to you. I hope you will like it. I am sure in the cold winter nights you will find it most useful.

I have had a great deal of surgery to do lately. I did an abdominal section about 3 weeks ago as a last resort to cure a patient, but she died 3 days after the operation from sheer exhaustion. So far as the operation was concerned I feel quite proud of it. I have to remove an Hydatid cyst from the lung when I return.

In referring to my last letter, it was not your brother who made the remarks at all — it was your mother, so I am to blame altogether and am sorry for being so hasty. I must thank you so much for the Piggy cards you sent me. Some of my patients have good laughs at them.

I must now close as I have only a few minutes to go to post and before doing so will tell you in a whisper that I like you now quite as much — which you never knew how much — as when we last parted.

Good bye and be good.
Your
Wm. C. Little

P.S. I send you views of Launceston and a book which may interest you.

Warracknabeal
April 13, 1893

My dear Grace

Your last letter, or volume, came to hand in due time and I was delighted to see it. What a jolly long letter. I think you have outstripped me this time. When I wrote you last I was in Tasmania where I spent a splendid holiday. I will not attempt to describe my travels as I think nearly everybody dabbles in more or less of the description of their travels. I went to Hobart, the capital of the Island. I visited many of the places you will see mentioned in that book I sent you, "Convict Life" by Nash. To tell you all about my wandering, the Mountains, gorges, the ravines, rivers, ferns would only spoil the picture, so I ask you just to imagine the most mountainous and rugged scenery and you will gain some idea of what I saw. I met some very nice people from England who were going the same round I was so I joined them and did enjoy their company and myself to my heart's content. The only inconvenience I felt from my sea voyage was I was always hungry. I could not get enough to eat. I had some fears that some ravenous disease or animal had taken possession of me so I hastened away to the scales & weighed myself and found I weighed 167 lbs. I concluded it was no fell disease but must be an animal, which after careful investigation I found to be correct and that ferocious animal was no less than myself. Oh, what a lovely thing it is to have a stomach that can digest huge big meals in about one to 1 ½ hrs and then crave for more. That was *MY* condition so I returned home fatter if not wiser and better than when I left. While on this eating subject, which is dear to everyone's heart, I must tell you a joke. I went to the Zoological Gardens in Sydney, N.S.W. I began to feel the pangs of hunger coming on again, so I hastened to an eating house where I saw Quong Tart stuck up in large letters. The waiter enquired what I would have so I said I would have a piece of Quong Tart as I had never heard of such a tart before. The waiter looked at me and I at him when he quietly informed me Quong Tart was the name of a very wealthy Chinaman who owned the premises as well as 20 more such institutions and that he is one of the wealthiest men in Sydney!

So much for Chinamen. By the way, I met Quong Tart afterwards and found him to be a very intelligent man.

While in Tasmania I came across a nice little possum rug which I thought you might like to have during the cold winter nights so I bought and sent it you by Tait's Express. It will go by England so it will [be] some

60 days before you receive it. You will see it about July 1st, or a little earlier. Kindly let me know when you see it as I have it insured against loss. I hope you will be good enough to accept it from me. It will be nice to put over the rocking chair or for you to curl upon on the sofa. It is nicer than the other one. I did not know how to send it until I was informed in Melbourne about Tait's Express.

My cousin, Dr. Cross, has gone home or at least he goes on the same boat as this letter will. I do not know whether he will be in Montreal or not. I shall give him your address and will ask him to call on you, should he go as far East. You will like him I know. He is nothing like his cheeky brother who is now in Africa eating negros.

I am glad you liked that photo and the beautiful home I have scattered around me.

Do you intend taking a holiday this summer? If so and you think of going to Toronto, I shall give you an invitation to visit my people when my sisters will plan a nice holiday in the backwoods of Muskoka where you can catch fish by the basketfulls. My people live in a very nice part of the city, 21 Division St., Toronto.

I was almost tempted to go to Chicago Exhibition but I couldn't go now if I wanted to. The Bank I was dealing with has gone "Crook" with $3000 of my money in it. However, I don't care much as it will right itself in two months and there then will not be a stronger bank on this side of the globe.

I had made arrangements to put it all out in land, had written the cheques etc. when the suspension came. It has done me good, it has sharpened me a bit. Two weeks ago I had not $5. I have since collected $700 and am not going to stop until I collect $5000 which is owing to me, so I am glad of what has happened. It is known for a certainty now that depositors will not lose a penny.

So much for financial matters. Well, I hope you got through your lecture on Hygiene and Dress. Do you purpose doing away with the corset, or not?

If you were as nervous as you say then you would prepare and deliver a good lecture. The more anxious I am about anything the more likely I am to succeed. Glad you have got into practice so nicely and that you get confinements occasionally. You will very soon get over that anxiety. I have reached the stage that I wish I could do without confinements. If you accept that offer I made you I will be most happy to let you attend them all. It is the hardest and worst paid work we do. The fees here $15-$30.

The beautiful silk handkerchief came to hand along with your letter and so allow me to tell you I like it so much. The "L" you worked on it is most beautifully done. It has been admired by several of my friends. I am saving it for special occasions when I shall show it off to the best advantage. How ancient I am getting to be — 33 last birthday. It is not difficult to remember my birthday. I cannot remember birthdays unless they come on some crazy day like my own. I am just about old enough to get married I guess, but I have a theory — there is nothing like having a theory — and that is Drs. and priests should never marry. Their lives should be devoted to bodily ailments and soul ailments.

I think I told you my brother is married. He has a nice home and a fat wife so he should be happy and warm during the winter. I wouldn't get married and bring a wife to this place for anything. As soon as I make enough money to take life easier I shall get out of this place, and travel awhile. As Byron [in] "The Ocean" says:

"There is a pleasure in the pathless wood
There is a rapture on the lonely shore" (ch. 7)

I shall tempt the ocean again but I don't think I was ever born to be drowned.

Mr. Wm. Fair's sister Mary — Mrs. Cockhill — died in confinement some two months ago.

Now Grace, good bye, and write me another long letter. It is like a kiss, all I can say is do it again. Your letters always give me hours of pleasure, so I hope they will continue. Kind regards to Mrs. Savage and your mother.

Sincerely yours,
Wm. C. Little

Warracknabeal
June 8, 1893.

My dear Grace,

I had intended beginning this letter yesterday in order that I would have heaps of time but professional calls kept me busy until late in the night. I am answering two letters this time as I was called in consultation some 30 miles when I should have answered the letter before the last. I did not get home until it was too late to catch the mail. The case I was called to was Purpura Hemorrhagica, the first case I ever saw in my life. I had no difficulty diagnosing it. The Dr. who was in attendance did not know what it was. Blood was extravasated in patches all over the legs — there was continuous hemorrhage from the nose and kidneys. I do not know when I met a more touching sight. The patient, a proud & noble man, President of a Shire — a man who had educated himself in every branch including classics. The poor man looked at me when I arrived as much as to say, "You will save me." Two helpless Drs. stood beside the patient's bed — we simply could do nothing. I merely mention this case in case you should meet one like it.

Well, I really forget where I left off the last time I wrote you. Life is pretty much of a sameness with me, with here and there bright spots in the way of surgical operations or the pleasure of meeting some new disease that I have had little experience in. I am called out, so will stop for a while. I have just returned from seeing a case of Graves' disease — the 2nd case I have seen in the Colony. There is no enlargement of the Thyroid but the eyes are protruding out of their sockets & the heart is running around 140 per minute, etc.

I have just had a big feed of mushrooms & some splendid fish for dinner so I should either become sleepy or be in the best of humor — well, I feel pretty well satisfied with myself which is always a pleasing thing to me. Let me see — what did Miss Abbott mean by writing that she could tell me something about you that would please me? Now Grace, you know we were not to keep any secrets from each other and there you have something stowed away possibly up the sleeve of your frock or elsewhere, the knowledge of which would please me — ha! ha! I have to laugh — What is it? — a new tooth where I pulled one out or is it an only recently discovered dimple on some part of your body which omens all kinds of good luck. Lord have mercy on my indolent brain, I cannot guess. I shall try again in all seriousness and I may succeed in guessing. Are you getting fat or thin or have you got a new sealskin jacket or are you the same jolly girl you were when I knew

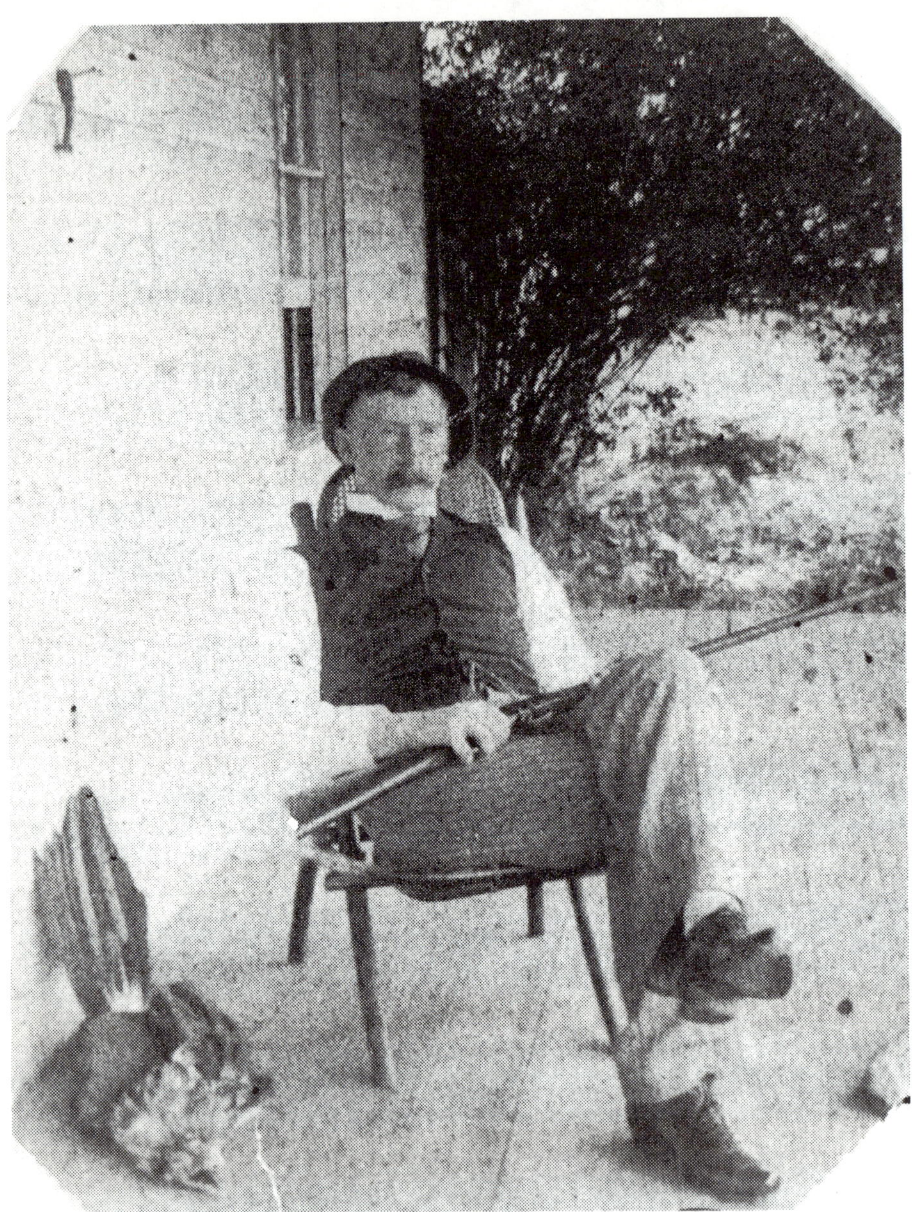

"Taken by an amateur away back in this wild woods as I had returned from shooting. The game you see is an old eagle head and tail & the body is made up of a bunch of rags — very good effect. When shooting that day I shot a swan, broke its wing, caught the swan & set its wing & let it go. I also shot an eagle & a big lizard, hence the self-satisfied expression on my sunburned face"

Billy's note on the back of the snapshot opposite

you or have you got big and stout with a hideous bonnet on the back of your head and all sorts of surgical expressions beaming from your face? Well, these are things not to dwell on as the man said when he sat down on some tacks and the lovers said when they sat down on an ants' nest. I shall write a reply to Miss Abbott's missive which, will you be kind enough to give her?

I shall have to give it up as I am no good at guessing. If I had your hand for a while I am positive as God made little apples that I could tell you the secret — or if you send me a model of it I am willing to wager $10 to $1 that I can tell you.

I most sincerely wish that your life is as comfortable and happy as you could possibly wish and in no way troubled by unkindly circumstances of fortune. These at least would give me the most pleasurable news I could hear of you.

Dingle goes the bell — A young man with three of his toes nearly cut off. I have stitched them on in the hope that they will grow on all right.

What a varied life a Dr. has. A Dr. requires to be Jack of all trades. I have stood Godfather for a child, have baptised two children in the Catholic faith, have drawn up agreements, wills, etc. I attended a dance one night, was called to a confinement after having a few dances, child was born in ½ an hour, was then called to a death bed and returned to the dance in time for the Highland Schottische and a waltz. Did you ever hear of such a mixture? I get the Bank to collect government accounts for me for P.Ms. etc. I called the other day for my banker to collect for me and he wanted to know what the money was for. I told him a couple of lunatics and a dead man. I thought the banker would have taken a fit. I seem to be on the horrible strain tonight. I feel as if live ghosts were wandering around.

I have been learning to play Solo whist lately. I am becoming pretty good at the game. It is the best game in cards I have played. It takes my mind completely off my work and rests my brain. You told me in one of your letters that you were a good card player. If you don't know Solo whist, learn it by all means and I shall put you to the test when I go home.

I have been getting a good deal of praise lately over some surgical performances. A young man received a kick over the right eye completely smashing in the frontal bone. I reflected the scalp and removed the smashed bone, some of which was driven into the brain. I elevated what pieces I could in the hope of union. Considerable quantities of brain escaped and one meningeal artery was cut. The surface of the brain exposed was the size of this diagram. I put a drainage tube into the brain, stitched up the scalp, gave grn.xv of Hyd. Sul. Chlor. and grn. xx pulv. Jalap sec. — followed by grn. xxx Pot.-Brom. The patient slowly and progressively recovered. I mail you a photo of Nurses of Hospital and the brain case sitting in a chair. The little girl in the photo had been treated for some 12 mos. for all sorts of things when I was called in to see her & diagnosed Pott's disease[56] of the spine — placed her in plaster of Paris jacket and had the pleasure of seeing her able to walk about, perfectly cured in 5 months. The nurse you see standing in the door is the best trained nurse I have met in my medical experience. The young woman standing beside the brain case is an assistant, the elderly lady is the matron. Unfortunately, I could not be present in the group.

I did a strabismus operation some two weeks ago. I am going to do an Iridectomy shortly. I don't believe in sending good cases to specialists. I do all kinds of operations on the bodies of patients who die in the hospital. In every case I do Chalazion operations and iridectomies so that I am becoming quite familiar with eye work. I shall be delighted when I can give up midwifery. I have had so much of it. I feel I have very little more to learn, besides, so many cases are normal and any old woman could do as well as I. I did an operation on the knee joint last Saturday. I opened the joint right up & removed a loose cartilage. The patient is doing beautifully. I must say it was a bit risky opening a large joint, however luck has been in my way.

Kindly let me know if you received a letter from me when I was in Tasmania. I think you should have received it before you wrote last time. I sent you some views of Launceston, also a book.

I hope you receive the opossum rug all right. I am sorry I did not send it earlier. However, it will come in good next winter.

I wish you every success in getting the hospital appointment, you will find you will gain any amount of practical experience. It will give you that confidence in yourself that is really necessary to secure the confidence of your patients. I have every confidence that you will get the appointment. I think your chart I gave you will indicate that your star is in the ascendency. Oh, that chart! Made up of all kinds of nonsense at the same time a vein of truth running through it. If you don't succeed don't blame the chart — blame yourself for you can accomplish anything in reason that you attempt.

It is nearly 12 o'clock so I must wind up and go down to the post office. I am going to cut some of the photo so I can get it into an envelope.

Kindly remember me to the Menagerie when you write to *it*.

My cousin Dr. Cross is at present in Canada with his wife and little boy. I do not think he will be in Montreal. He is only going to be away 6 mos., the greater part of his visit will be spent in Chicago and the northwest.

When I look over what I have written I feel sensible that it is a poor miserable scrawl. I know you will be good enough to overlook what you may see amiss. I am delighted to receive your letters and to know you are prospering.

I remain sincerely yours,
W.C. Little

P.S. I have given Miss Abbott a conundrum. Do tell me what she says about my note.

P.S. 2 — I have a crematory day once every three months in which all answered correspondence is committed to the flames in the hope of a glorious resurrection!

Warracknabeal
October 24, 1893

My dear Grace,

I know well that you will have me put away in the back of your book as I did not answer your last letter. I intended writing but mail time went by and as you were going to Chicago I concluded you would hear & see quite enough without being bothered reading my uninteresting letters. I received your letter of Sept. 12th; altho' brief, it gave a great deal of information. I am so sorry my people were away from home when you called. My father and one of my sisters were away to Chicago — possibly you met them. My mother and sisters — the balance of them — were away upon the Muskoka lakes fishing and enjoying themselves to their hearts' content.

My sisters were very sorry to have missed meeting you — of course I have told them a good deal about you and how clever you are so they have a very great respect for you and would be most pleased to meet you. Your card was found in letter box or under the door. My sister Lizzie who is married in Nova Scotia and my sister, Bella,[57] will be passing through Montreal and if time will allow of it, will call on you. Thanks so much for the "Journal" with beautiful views of Chicago Exhibition. I am reading it whenever I have a spare moment. I have shown the views to a good many and they had no idea that such a magnificent building would be put up to be pulled down again.

Life with me is just the same week after week and month after month, with an occasional break in its monotony with a good operation or a holiday. I have been using the knife pretty freely lately. I had a gory week of it recently. Mention of some of it was much in the local papers. which I shall cut out and enclose in this letter. A German Dr. and I removed a kidney successfully and patient is doing well, going on to complete recovery. The kidney was very adherent, however with care & patience we succeeded in breaking them down with little if any injury to the peritoneum. There was a good deal of peritoneal irritation afterwards but that was controlled all right.

I am slowly and gradually getting a name as a surgeon. I think my next operation of note will be an ovarian cystic tumor. The patient says she will not allow any other Dr. to touch her. Do not think that I am getting conceited. I may be, but I do not think so. I consider I am fortunate and have the knack of making people believe in me. I have every confidence in myself, which may be conceit or ignorance or competency. I shall endeavour not to get too fat. I am in good condition for the summer which is just coming

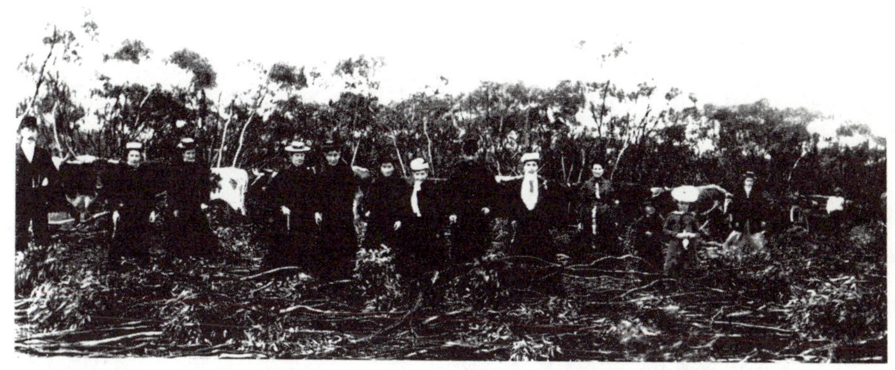

Dr. Little (L) and friends clearing the scrub

on. I am pleased to tell you that I am not bald headed and [have] not the slightest symptoms of it coming on as I have a better crop of hair than ever I had.

I am glad you at last have got a fixed place of abode and likely to stay awhile. I think changing residence interferes with your practice, particularly in the early stages. Hope your Chinese patient still sticks to you.

I am still dabbling a little in speculation. I bought a farm of 320 acres a few days ago for $3000 cash. I expect to get $4500 for it on terms $1000 down, the balance in one two and three years and 7% for my money. It amuses me to hear people talk about my luck — the truth is, I know more about business matters than I choose to let on. I always say, "I don't know anything about business." I landed a lawyer over the land transaction to the tune of $100 — He thought I was anxious to get the land — it was sold by auction — and as the estate owed him money, it occurred to him that it would be a good time to run me for it. He bid once too often and the land was knocked down to the poor devil. I took the precaution before the sale to have the contract of sale strictly cash — Mr. Lawyer couldn't pay for it so I got it at my own bid and he had to pay the difference. I informed him while he thought he had all the brains in the town he didn't put them to profitable use. This is the second time I have landed him for his conceit.

I invited some of my friends to take a trip out into the country to see how land is cleared of scrub, how plowing is done etc. I took a photographer with me and we were taken. I shall send you a photo but I fear I cannot get one in time for this mail.

I have sent my winter horses out to grass and I have got my lovely ponies in for the summer work. I took some prizes with my horses as you will see by a clipping enclosed — got $20 in prizes for my horses. I would have taken 1st for everything only one of the horses that I was having schooled over high jumps hurt his leg and it was a little swollen. I hope for better luck next time.

Evidently you did not look up Dr. McGrath when you were in Chicago — You know he was one of your admirers in Kingston. I wonder how he is getting on? I am such a bad correspondent. I lose track of my fellow graduates.

I was surprised to notice in the last Royal Calendar that Dr. Henderson is *dead*. I wonder what he died of — I am really curious about him as he appeared to be a man of robust physique. Kindly let me know if you hear any particulars.

I notice Dr. Norman Grant, a fellow graduate, is practising in New Zealand. Should everything turn out as I have planned, I shall look him up next March as I purpose going there for my holiday. I am glad to hear Miss Henderson is doing well. If I had known she was going to Hamilton I would have sent a letter of introduction to Dr. Stormes, a particular friend of mine. I have not decided when I shall take a trip home. So long as my parents are reported to be in good health, I keep putting [it] off. I cannot leave here easily as I am going up up up and it would be unwise for me to go away for such a time. When people think they are tired of me, if I go away for 6 mos., they will welcome me back — at least that is my reading of human nature.

I think I wrote Miss Abbott a rather impertinent note for which I am sorry. I did it on the spur of the moment. I hope she does not think me rude.

Now Grace, good bye and be *good* as my mother and sisters used to say to me & altho I am a bad correspondent I assure you your letters give me the greatest pleasure I get out of this kangaroo country.

Sincerely yours as ever,
Wm. C. Little

Melbourne
March 16, 1894

My dear Grace

Once more I am on terra solid — have just returned from my New Zealand trip and I find the Canadian mail goes out tomorrow morning. I am in a bit of a quandary to know just where to begin this letter. I am at a loss to know what I have told you and have not. However, I am alive, living, fat, strong, robust, with my hair on and almost *good looking*. "Vanity of vanities," saith the preacher. I shall refer to my *good looks* later on without consulting the preacher.

In my last letter I told you how ill I had been with typhoid which you were aware of before I wrote. You see, even in my delirium I did not forget you as I told my brother to write to you. I did not read your letter for two weeks afterwards. I tried to but could not concentrate my mind. My nurse after a fortnight allowed me to read one page at a time. I do hope you are well and that you may never get typhoid fever or the measles.

So soon as I got strong enough to hobble about, I came to Melbourne where I remained ½ a day and a night. Then I took passage to New Zealand. I was scarcely able to walk on the boat. I was so thin you could have read a newspaper through me. Now after a three weeks' trip I am all I have told you on first page. Referring to good looking, my face has got quite fat. All the wrinkles filled up, a good fresh color too due to the fact that the greater part of my present flesh is young, *succulent* and of the baby type or embryonic i.e., not fully developed. I could almost tie a knot in my legs before I left; now I am so fat I can scarcely cross them. Fancy me writing you such horrible things. I should have said "extremities" not "legs" — when you write "legs" you naturally think of the dissecting room or the ballet, where those things were not covered with a super abundance of clothing.

I think I told you what pleasure it gave me to use profane language after my recovery. I could swear all the time and I found it did me good, possibly I was getting rid of the microbes. This suggests an idea that it might be possible that all bad morality may be due to those little brats of microbes. If such should turn out to be a truth, what a revolution would take place in the Ecclesiastical persuasion. Well, I am now a respectable citizen, & do not use bad words; in fact, I say a prayer every morning, viz. "Thank God I am alive to see such lovely things and not to be a bit sea sick, etc." I am enjoying life I believe better than I did before I was ill.

A little over 3 weeks ago I sailed for New Zealand, calling at Hobart in Tasmania where I spent 24 hours — from thence to the beautiful New Zealand South, thence to the Bluff, Invercargill, Port Chalmers, Dunedin, Port Lyttletown, Christ-Church, Wellington, Napier, Auckland, etc. and I had from 24 to 60 hours in each of those places so that I got a pretty good idea of the New Z. cities. I returned via Sydney. If you look on a map you will at once see I had a good long trip. I met and conversed with lots of Maories. I did not fall in love with any of them. Fancy kissing a tattooed Maori. The Maori women tattoo their upper lips and lower ones also & they look horrid. I would as soon kiss a goat. The half-castes are rather pretty, their eyes being their charm. Unfortunately they do not live long as they seem very susceptible to phthisis.

There is no use me attempting to describe the scenery for I could not do it as my vocabulary does not contain enough of superlative adjectives to give you any idea of the beauty, magnificence and gorgeous grandeur of the scenery back in Tasmania & New Zealand.

Let me see — your birthday has gone by and I did not send you even a card. How horrid of me. I have always been deficient in what I might call the little courtesies which go to make our lives a wee bit brighter and happier in the remembering of birthdays, Xmas, New Year and Easter. I shall soon be another year older, beautiful 34 and still a bachelor. Well, well and so it will continue to the end of the chapter for all I know.

I expect some letters to be forwarded tomorrow when I expect to see one from you. I do not resume practice for a fortnight yet. I am going in the hill country to hunt Kangaroos on horseback. The exercise will strengthen and harden my soft muscles.

I expected to be sailing for home in about a month had I not been ill and my father's little troubles come in the way. Better luck next time is my prayer.

Now good bye and may you always be happy is my wish.

Sincerely
William C. Little

"And So They Lived…"

"And So They Lived..."

It is impossible to believe that the closing words of the last letter (March 16, 1894) were really the last that Billy Little ever wrote to Grace Ritchie. In themselves, removed from the context of the rest of the letter, the words "Now goodbye and may you always be happy is my wish" do strike a note of finality. There is a touch of sadness about them, too, so that on reading them it is easy enough to think of him riding off romantically into the sunset. In reality, he was probably just in the Dandenongs relaxing and recuperating from the terrible typhoid fever, fully expecting to return to Warracknabeal, eagerly anticipating a letter from her the following day, confident of continuing the correspondence.

Did her letter come? What did it say?

It is true that the frequency and length of his letters had flagged because of his ill-health and because the memories of 1888–1889, their year together, were becoming overlaid by time, distance, and diverging interests. Once he had fretted, "It is awfully hard to write a whole souled letter sometimes, isn't it? Do you know, I fancy you do, that I cannot write you as good a letter now as I could a year ago . . . because I have not been in your company for such a long time . . ." (November 23, 1890). And she apparently felt they were becoming "strangers to each other" (March 20, 1891). There may also be some significance to the fact that she stopped noting when she received and answered his letters. All the same, he showed no signs of forsaking her, telling her that "your letters add a bright thread to the web of my life" (August 3, 1890) and more recently (October 24, 1893) had reassured her that they gave him the "greatest of pleasure I get out of this kangaroo country." He swore that "even in his delirium" he had not forgotten her. Indeed, his more recent letters reveal greater emotion than the earlier ones. What then happened? Did he "continue to the end of the chapter" still a bachelor as he was in mid-March, 1894, when he contemplated his forthcoming birthday? Did he ever return to Canada? What kind of career did he ultimately have? Did he continue to do as well professionally and financially as he began? What of her? Did the parallel lines ever converge?

There are none of William C. Little's letters to answer these or the host of other questions that come to mind. Further letters must have existed, but either Grace Ritchie did not keep them, or they were lost or burned. The rest of the story must, perforce, be pieced together from other sources — newspapers, his obituary, his will, her papers, fragile memories.

We have to rely merely on conjecture to assume that not so very long after W.C.L. returned to Warracknabeal he did receive a letter from Grace Ritchie. Perhaps it told him, "Come home at once or else, . . ." and he was unable to accept her ultimatum. Perhaps it simply told him there was no use in coming back because she intended to marry Dr. Frank England of Montreal.

Marry Frank England she did. The wedding took place in April, 1897, and the news of that event, whenever or however it came to Billy Little not only would have shattered his hopes regarding her, but also undermined his resolve to return to Canada. We now know for sure that he remained a resident of Warracknabeal and that he never married; we are certain that his career continued in Australia, hers in Canada.

○   ○   ○

When she received that last letter of March 16, 1894, Grace Ritchie had already graduated in medicine. She had transferred from the Kingston Women's Medical College to Bishop's College because the latter had offered her a place in its Faculty of Medicine in Montreal. Amid a class of men, she was more than ever determined to succeed. She came first in the final examination and, when she was awarded the Bishop's C.M., M.D. in 1891, she became the first woman in the province of Quebec to receive a medical degree. In the approved manner of the day, Dr. Ritchie then went to Europe for post-graduate work in Glasgow, Paris, and Vienna. Neither her earnestness nor the presence of her mother seemed to prevent her from attracting the gallantries of several gentlemen. She also won the praises of the distinguished physicians with whom she studied in Vienna.

When she returned to Montreal she still had to face the old prejudice against lady doctors, but she was well-supported by her excellent credentials and again she broke new ground. She was one of the first women to receive a medical licence in Quebec and to set up a private practice. That was not all. She was given a position as demonstrator in anatomy at Bishop's; the only woman ever to be taken onto the staff of its medical faculty. She turned down an offer of a job as house surgeon in a private hospital, but accepted an appointment as assistant gynaecologist at the Western Hospital in Montreal. In both of her appointments she had special responsibility for women. This must have pleased her for, while she was proving herself, she was furthering the cause of women.

One winter's day, Dr. Ritchie received a letter, not from afar, but from someone close at hand. It said in a very straightforward way:

58 Beaver Hall Hill
Montreal

Feby 2nd

Dear Dr. Ritchie

I am obliged to drive to Montreal Junction this afternoon and would like very much to have you go with me. Can it be arranged? If convenient for you, I will call, say at 4.45 o'clock; we would then arrive home in time for dinner.

Yours sincerely,
F.R. England

If tomorrow would suit you better, I could postpone trip till then. Telephone between 2 & 3.

Dr. Frank Richardson England, the writer of this letter, was just five years older than Grace Ritchie. He was a Montreal surgeon and a lecturer at Bishop's, and she had been in one of his classes. He considered her to have been his most talented student. While he was also recognized as brilliant, he evoked sympathy as well as respect because his wife had recently died, leaving him with a four-year-old son, Murray, to raise. Through 1895 and 1896, Dr. England wrote Dr. Ritchie increasingly personal letters, saw her as frequently as possible and, finally, it was he whom she chose to marry.

The *Montreal Daily Star* of April 6, 1897, described the wedding as "a quiet one," noting that only relatives were present but that "the church was prettily decorated with white cut flowers and palms." After the ceremony, the bride wore "a smart tailor-made going-away gown of ashes of roses cloth. The skirt and short coat were of the cloth, the coat opening over a pink and rose checked silk shirt waist. Her hat was of rose and green straw, with

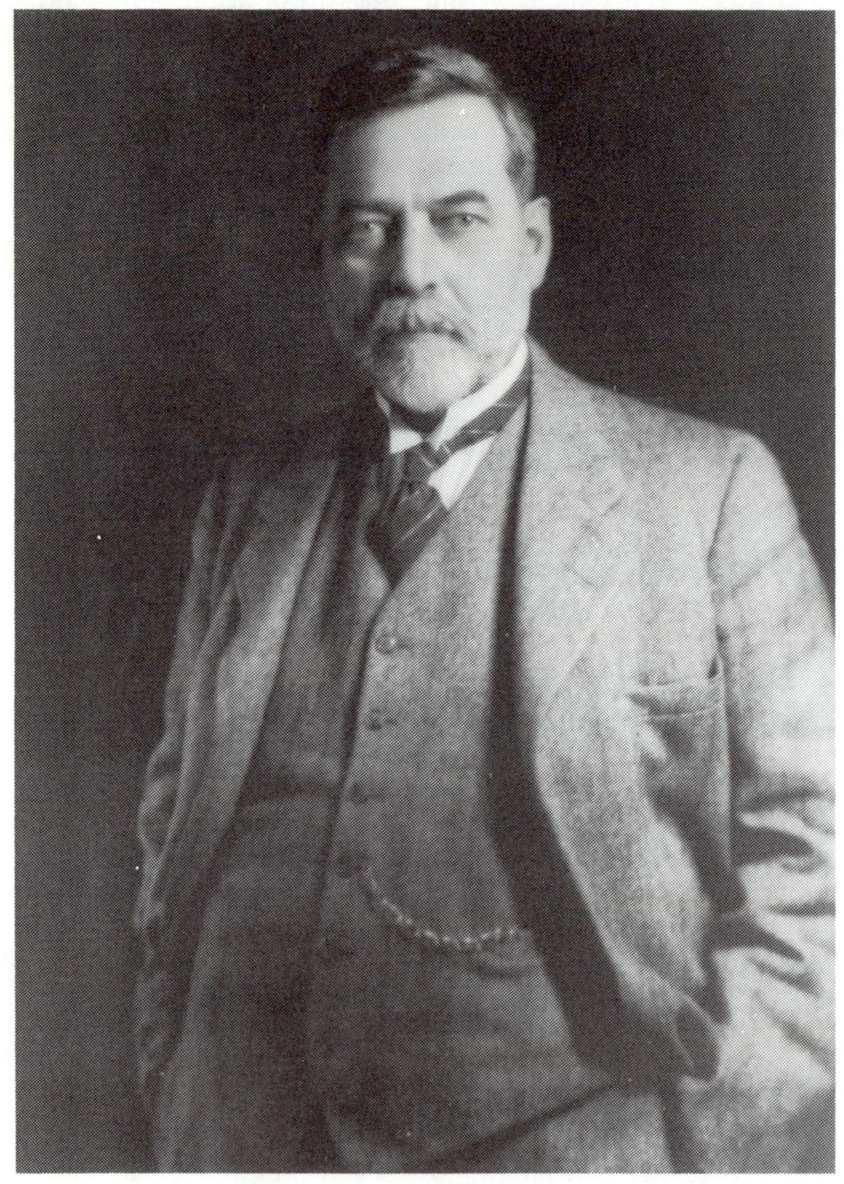

Dr. Frank Richardson England.

pink chiffon and aigrette of bright green grass. She carried a large bouquet of white roses, the gift of the groom." The happy couple spent their honeymoon travelling extensively in Europe and returned to Montreal in September.

Henceforth, Grace was known as Dr. Ritchie-England; marriage did not interfere unduly with her career. Not for her an immediate retirement. Although she had resigned from Bishop's in April, 1896 (a year before the wedding), she stayed on at the Western Hospital for another decade, retiring about seven months *after* the birth of her only daughter, Esther. In accepting her resignation, the hospital's medical board expressed its high opinion of her contribution, observing that:

> Her work as Assistant-Gynaecologist will long be remembered for its thoroughness and the large attendance attracted to her clinic. Her name will always be connected with the creation of the present system of Hospital case reporting and statistics, upon which the improved Annual Medical Reports for some years past have been based. [1]

The board of governors also placed on record its appreciation of the valuable and faithful services rendered, noting that the "clinic presided over by her for the past thirteen years was one of the most efficiently cared for in the Out Patient Dept. of the Hospital." [2]

The withdrawal from the hospital ended a phase of Grace Ritchie-England's career, but certainly not her public life. For many years she continued her own medical practice, "ministering to women who find it best to consult a sympathetic woman physician, both counsellor and friend." [3] Like many other medical women of her time, she became very much involved in social issues. This was not a new, but an ongoing concern for her. Ever since her student days she had championed the rights of women. Now, despite the demands first of medicine and then of family, she remained active in organizations supporting causes such as the female franchise, child health, compulsory education, and legal reform. Energetic, forthright, prominent, she was chosen to represent Canada at several international conferences and was paticularly involved with women's groups. In 1896 she began a long association with the Montreal Local Council of Women, later became a member of the National Council, and ultimately, of the International Council of Women. Her visit to Rome in 1914 to attend the International Council meeting was recalled seventy years later by her daughter:

> The Presidents of various Local Councils were entertained by Italy's Queen Margarita, who was a Montenegran princess before her marriage. The Queen entertained the ladies graciously and presented representatives with bouquets of

roses. Each bouquet had a silver medal with insignia attached. Some kind person told the Queen that Mother had a small daughter with her and she very kindly gave Mother another bunch, saying, "For your little girl." No wonder I was very thrilled to be given a present from a real queen.[4]

From 1912 to 1918, Dr. Grace Ritchie-England served as president of the Local Council of Women. Her dynamic leadership was put to effective use in organizing war-time causes such as a hospital ship fund, the collection of furs for troops serving in the Alps, the Serbian Relief Fund, the Patriotic Fund and the Red Cross. The tributes she received from the women of Montreal when she stepped down were much more significant than the usual plaudits accorded retiring presidents of voluntary organizations. They were more like public apologies, amends she richly deserved. For the last several months of her six-year term had been fraught with drama and controversy that might have broken a lesser woman.

In the highly contentious federal election campaign of 1917, Dr. Grace Ritchie-England created a furore when she endorsed Sir Wilfrid Laurier and openly criticized the Union Government under Sir Robert Borden. Not one to mince words, she called Borden's regime "moribund, discredited and unrepresentative."[5] At issue were two pieces of legislation: the Military Service Act, which introduced conscription, but that she condemned as "utterly failing to provide the necessary reinforcements for our men at the front" because of the unfair exemptions it made; and the War-Times Election Act, which gave the federal vote to women for the first time, but only to those women who were in the armed forces or who were relatives of military men. This she considered a piece of "unsurpassed effrontery which sets at defiance every fundamental of British justice" because selected women were enfranchised only in the expectation that they would vote for conscription.

Grace Ritchie-England's penetrating, outspoken views proved unpopular with many of the fervidly patriotic club women of her city. Her objections were completely misinterpreted and she was accused of being unsympathetic to the war effort. The Montreal Women's Club almost unanimously passed a resolution demanding her resignation as president of the Local Council of Women on the grounds that as president she should not be taking part in politics and because she was "opposing the immediate sending of reinforcements to our brave boys in France."[6] This became front-page news, especially when the Montreal Women's Club executive resigned in an elaborate show of support for her. Regardless of this gesture, she was privately shunned as well as publicly ridiculed. She suffered much anguish and what she called "a small measure of persecution." In the end, her friends

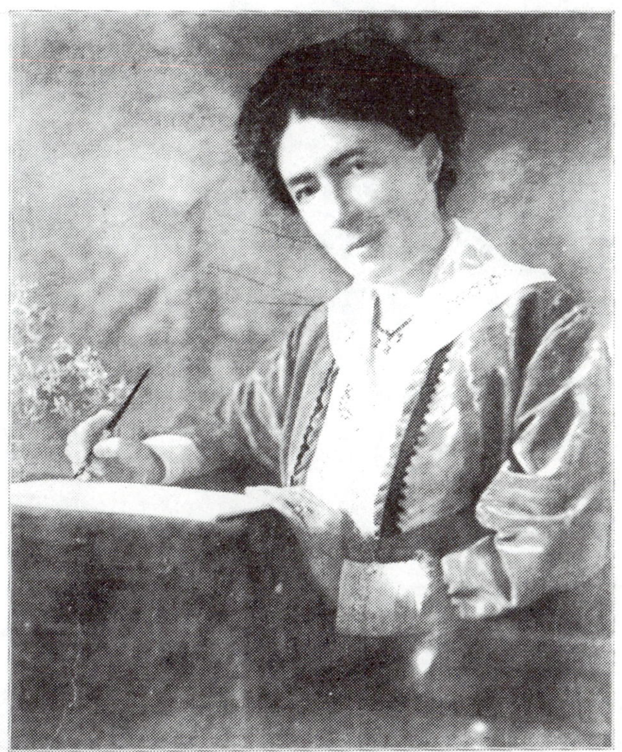

Grace Ritchie as the first female Liberal Party candidate

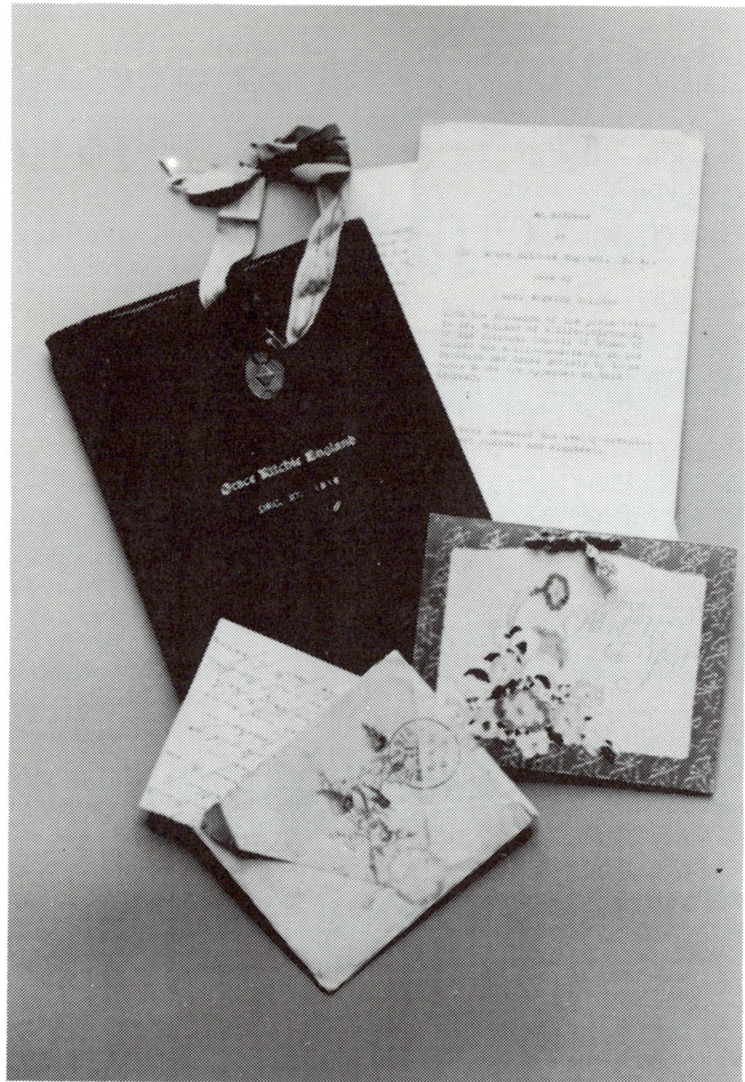

Tributes to Dr. Grace Ritchie-England

and those who could see the integrity of her position restored the balance. She was fêted at the Ritz, presented with a life patronage of the National Council of Women, a life membership of the Canadian Red Cross Society, and given a copy of a glowing accolade signed by 136 of Montreal's most distinguished women. This acknowledged that:

> During the tumult of war and consequent national effort, it
> was easy to neglect the nearer patriotism, although in it were
> involved the same principles as those so dearly paid for on
> European battle fields. But some there were who saw with
> true vision the interrelation between the war for democratic
> ideals and the maintenance of those ideals at home . . . .[7]

Her fellow club members also made it clear that they considered her "a
national asset," and praised her for maintaining "her poise through trying
times" and made their presentation as an expression of their "admiration,
esteem and affection."

At heart, Grace Ritchie-England was a gentle person, but she gave
some militant advice to her successor as president of the Local Council of
Women: "In spite of discouragement, stick to your guns." That is what she
herself always did and even the searing experience in the Council did not
deter her from further public work or from charting new courses. After the
federal franchise was granted to all Canadian women in 1918, she kept working
with suffragists like Thérèse Casgrain for the right of women to vote in the
province of Quebec. They finally won, but not until 1940. Meanwhile, in
1930, Dr. Ritchie-England became the first woman to stand for federal parliament as an endorsed candidate of the Liberal Party of Canada. She did not
win against her entrenched Conservative opponent — she had not expected
to — but she gave him a scare and said she was satisfied to have paved the
way for other women. "It is a beginning . . . ,"[8] she said. And so it was.

Grace Ritchie's life seems to have been very successful and happy.
Her relationship with Frank England was infused with understanding and
affection, and both of them were devoted to Esther, their "D.D." or Darling Daughter. Dr. Ritchie-England's vitality never seemed to flag, though
after her husband's death in 1942, she slowed down a little. In her later years
she spent more time in the Eastern Townships, where she had built a charming
summer home at Knowlton and created an enviable garden out of a rocky
field. When she died on February 1, 1948, tributes poured in from all over
Canada. Her many friends praised the personal qualities of this warm,
magnetic, many-talented woman; while the prime minister himself lauded
her contribution to public life. Grace Ritchie became a person of prominence,
but there is no way of knowing how much thought she gave during her busy
career to Billy Little, who had written to her so regularly so long ago, or
whether she ever heard from him again, or whether she ever had any regrets
for what might have been. "Well supposing . . ." (January 23, 1890).

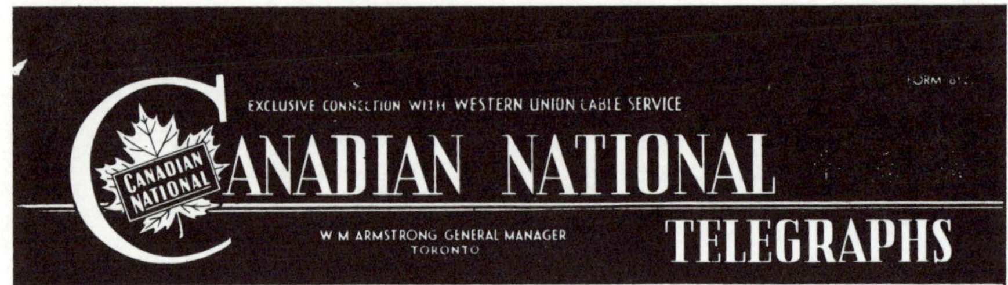

CANADIAN NATIONAL TELEGRAPHS

EXCLUSIVE CONNECTION WITH WESTERN UNION CABLE SERVICE

W M ARMSTRONG GENERAL MANAGER
TORONTO

STANDARD TIME

FEB 3 PM 5 54
(53)

GA278 117 DL=OTTAWA ONT 3 502P

MRS ERIC A CUSHING=

9 LORRAINE ST MTL=

=MY DEAR MRS CUSHING: I CANNOT EXPRESS TOO SINCERELY THE SYMPATHY I FEEL FOR YOU IN THE PASSING OF YOUR DEAR AND DISTINGUISHED MOTHER. AMONG CANADIAN WOMEN, DR. GRACE RITCHIE ENGLAND WAS MORE THAN OUTSTANDING. MEDICINE, EDUCATION, PUBLIC LIFE OWE MUCH TO HER EXCEPTIONAL ABILITIES AND NOBLE PUBLIC SPIRIT. THE LIBERAL PARTY IN CANADA IS ESPECIALLY INDEBTED TO HER FOR YEARS OF LEADERSHIP IN THE ADVANCEMENT OF LIBERAL PRINCIPLES AND POLICIES. AS LEADER OF THE LIBERAL PARTY, I SHARE YOUR LOSS IN THE PASSING OF ONE WHO, THROUGHOUT THE YEARS OF MY LEADERSHIP, WAS A DEVOTED PERSONAL FRIEND, AND, IN ALL THAT PERTAINED TO THE ADVANCEMENT OF THE PARTY'S PRINCIPLES AND POLICIES, AN ABLE AND LOYAL LIEUTENANT=

=W L MACKENZIE KING.

○ ○ ○

Billy Little's career was not as spectacular as Grace Ritchie's. He never became a national figure and no prime minister wired condolences at his death, yet he, too, held public office and his name was frequently in the newspapers. Soon after his arrival in Australia he became an honorary surgeon and later Senior Honorary Medical Officer at the Horsham Hospital; for many years he was District Health Officer and Vaccination Officer in Warracknabeal and, most important, he was elected Medical Officer at the Warracknabeal District Hospital. This hospital, which opened in 1891, was supported by some government grants but relied heavily on local subscriptions. Like other public hospitals in Victoria, it was intended particularly for those people who could not afford private medical care. In the usual way, it was administered by an elected committee of town and countrymen, with the Medical Officer having chief professional responsibility, especially for surgery, and the Matron being in charge of the nursing staff and day-to-day matters. By contemporary standards, the Warracknabeal hospital was small. Reports presented at the monthly committee meetings show that in the 1890s it had twelve beds, with an average daily number of ten in-patients and an annual total of about one hundred and fifty out-patients. The position of medical officer at first netted Dr. Little only £50 per annum. This was later doubled, but was still a relatively low stipend. Nevertheless, the position was an important one that distinguished him in his community. He was enormously pleased to have the appointment at the hospital and to be made Shire Health Officer.

In addition, Dr. Little had his private practice. This practice was a flourishing one, and he seemed more than pleased with the financial rewards. He was sure that he was prospering more quickly than he would have if he had been in Canada. Chances are that he was correct. Fees approved for Victoria in the late nineteenth century were higher than those established for Ontario. However, in both places there was a permissable range that doctors could charge for medical services, so that fee scales are not necessarily meaningful. It is also hard to make precise comparisons because, even after the exchange rates have been calculated and the fee scales examined, there would still be a host of variables in considering what his actual cost of living would have been. Happily, one thing is clear. The amounts he indicated in his letters were generally on the low side of the scale adopted by the medical profession for Victoria. It would be true to say that W.C.L. was enthusiastic about his income, but it could not be said that he was greedy.

He also had an interest in a private hospital that, to the puzzlement of the locals, he called "Massawippi." As his letters so clearly indicate, his practice involved many out-of-town calls and must have made heavy demands on his time and strength. Although he sometimes might have said, "Darn them, why don't they get sick in the day time?" (April 10, 1890), he seemed to rejoice in his work. Despite the remoteness of his location, he had not buried himself in the wilderness. He clearly wanted to keep up to date, continued to read, asked Grace to send him news of recent medical developments while she was in Europe, and he was ever willing to try new methods or to improvise as required. He seems to have had some remarkable successes with the use of hypnotism. This may have been relatively uncommon in the bush in the 1890s, but it was certainly not unknown in Australia then. As early as 1850, William Edwards had published, in Melbourne, a book called *Mesmerism: Its Practice and Phenomena.* This was basically an appeal to Australian doctors to use hypnotism more generally. It began:

> Mesmerism . . . is a Science of such vast importance and the result and benefits which would inevitably accrue from its universal adoption are so varied and so interesting, that one of the greatest wonders connected with it, is, that men of intellect and talent should continue to oppose it. . . . When it is taken out of the hands of the charlatan and placed in its legitimate sphere, viz: the medical profession, it will immediately assume its proper character and be generally acknowledged and adopted. (p. 9)

Dr. Little may or may not have read Edwards, but he had read other works and strongly favoured H. Bernheim's *Suggestive Therapeutics.* He assuredly also knew of the interest some Australian medical men were taking in hypnotism and spiritualism. While there were advertisements in the Melbourne newspapers that flirted with quackery, there were also publications on these subjects by respected physicians such as Walter Lindesay Richardson. Dr. Richardson, who had become, in 1869, the first president of the Victorian Association for Progressive Spiritualists, explained his participation in this field by his conviction that both it and hypnotism would be scientifically justified through observation and experiment.[9] The open-mindedness that allowed Dr. Little to try hypnotism, together with his concern for the welfare of his patients, brought him considerable wealth, along with much gratitude, respect, and affection. The gold thermometer and other gifts testify to this. So does the fact that the local newspapers made more frequent, positive and approving references to his activities than to those of any of his colleagues in the district. Stories about him were also handed down by word of mouth and, as late as 1983, Mrs. Winnie Leveire, Dr. Little's last known remaining patient, gratefully swore that he made superhuman efforts to save her from "inflammation of the brain" when she was an infant.

In brief, Dr. William C. Little proved that he was able, ambitious, and worthy of public appointment, so that his first decade in medicine was a story of increasing success and growing prominence. He might well have made an important mark on his profession. Yet his career suddenly changed course in 1901. What happened in Warracknabeal that year not only seriously affected Dr. Little's professional life, it also makes a fascinating case study of how local politics work in medicine.

○ ○ ○

In 1901, Dr. William C. Little had to face an unexpected series of crises. The events of that pivotal year, seen in retrospect, are framed by two apparently innocuous announcements in a local newspaper. The *Warracknabeal Herald,* in its issue of Friday, January 4, 1901, noted that:

> Dr. W.C. Little's many friends will be glad to learn that he is recovering from his illness, ptomaine poisoning, which on Tuesday was causing his friends considerable anxiety. The doctor last night had sufficiently gained strength to enable him to arrange for a holiday shortly . . .

The December 17 number said:

> Dr. W.C. Ross of Dimboola, who has not been in good health lately, intends taking a lengthy holiday.

These two trivial items might suggest nothing more than the general notion that medical practice in the country can be so rigorous that even doctors get sick or that doctors also need holidays. They hardly hint that there was a specific link between the careers of Dr. Little and Dr. Ross. In reality, there was an important connection and, because of it, there could be little doubt that both men would have sorely needed vacations. For both of them, that second year of the twentieth century must have caused considerable personal stress, as well as serious professional discomfort.

As the first news item cited above shows, 1901 did not begin well for William Little. He was ill. He probably got some kind of food poisoning during the Christmas/New Year festivities, a likely enough occurrence in the days before refrigeration and insecticides in a place where temperatures could hit the hundred mark and where country feasts would be well attended by flies and other pests. The *Herald,* which generally showed a sympathetic interest in Dr. Little's affairs, gave a running account of the state of his health: he began to improve but suffered a relapse on the following Sunday; a week later he was "sufficiently recovered to take outdoor exercise"; and he finally left for his holiday on January 18. He was away for about six weeks, returning to Warracknabeal in early March, having missed the worst of the dry, hot summer. He resumed his normal duties, feeling that the bad start to the year was behind him.

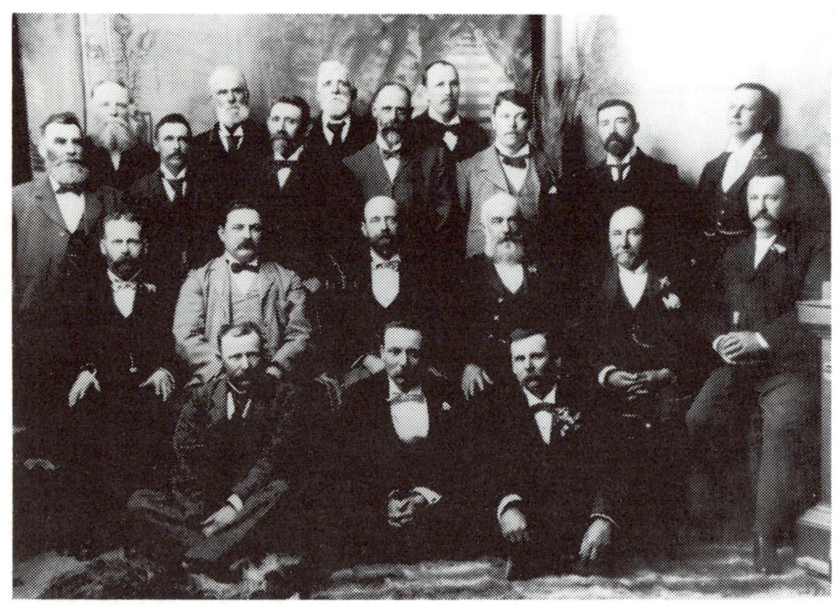

The Warracknabeal Hospital Committee, 1897. Mr. G. Miller is third from left in back row

Through the papers we then see glimpses of him as he announces that he would recommence vaccination (April 16), was reappointed honorary medical officer to the Ladies' Benevolent Society (July 12), attended patients with a variety of problems, successfully sued a wealthy patient who had neglected payment of bills amounting to £12.11.6. Usually, the *Herald*'s reports were simple statements of the fact that Dr. Little had been called to attend a man who had cut the top off his finger, or a woman who was badly burned, or a child who had been bitten by a snake, or a farmer who had been kicked by one of his animals. Occasionally, the paper injected a word of special approval as, for example, when it noted that Dr. Little had operated on a Hopetoun man who was badly crushed when a horse fell on him. It commented: "The man's life was despaired of, but under the skillful treatment of the doctor, his recovery has been marvellous" (March 12).

Things began to go wrong again for W.C.L. in June, when tensions began to develop between him and the Warracknabeal Hospital Committee.

The members of that committee also had a hectic year in 1901: they had to adjudicate an impertinent complaint by a nurse probationer against the hospital's matron; to supervise renovations because part of the hospital building had been condemned; to fill unexpected staff vacancies; to cope with allegations of religious bias; to organize a sports day and award prizes to the farmers who donated the most wheat; and, most important, they had to act in two serious medical cases. To some degree, both of these cases involved Dr. Little. Both also had political overtones.

The first case concerned an injured man called Jewitt who was brought to the hospital for emergency treatment following an accident on the Dimboola road, about two and-a-half miles from Warracknabeal. [10] The matron did not admit him, but told James Reed, who had taken Jewitt to the hospital, that the quickest way to get treatment would be to go directly to the medical officer's residence. Thus Jewitt was taken to Dr. Little's house. However, the matron said she expected him to be brought back to the hospital for admission. He did not appear and, a few days later, she learned that he had been admitted to Nurse Gaff's private hospital, the one in which Dr. Little had an interest.

This became a *cause célèbre*. Rumours spread throughout the district that Jewitt had been refused admission to the public hospital. The hospital committee was furious, since members were concerned for the reputation of the institution and worried that country people might withdraw their support. Dr. Little said that when Mr. Jewitt was brought to him, he had dressed his wound and, having no idea that he had already been taken to the public hospital and no indication that he wanted to go there, had sent him to Nurse Gaff's hospital.

The next meeting of the hospital committee was a highly charged affair. A committeeman called G. Miller declared that James Reed had told Dr. Little that Jewitt had already been to the hospital and that the matron had refused treatment. Other evidence was given that the matron had telephoned Dr. Little to say the patient was on his way. This the matron denied. Yet it was she who bore the brunt of the committeemen's anger. They passed a resolution that she and all members of the hospital staff should be fully aware of the admissions policy:

> Members of the Committee and honorary professional staff
> shall have a discretionary power of recommending in-patients
> and outpatients, *subject to the approval of the committee.*
> Accidents and cases of decided emergency shall be admitted
> at any time . . . ,

They also set up a formal investigation into this matter, which they considered to be a serious one. The matron was reprimanded, and she and one of the nurses subsequently resigned. That, however, was not the end of the affair. Indeed, it seemed to provide an opportunity for an opening gambit against Dr. Little.

During the July meeting, Mr. Miller raised the issue of what we today might call "conflict of interest," but that he termed "the advisability of the Medical Officer of the public hospital being connected with private hospitals." He gave notice of a motion stating that it was "not conducive to the best interests of the public hospital" for the medical officer to have any interest, direct or indirect, in a private hospital. Further, the motion called for the termination within three months of Dr. Little's engagement as medical officer. New applications were to be called for and it was to be stipulated that the medical officer should not be interested in any private institution, that he should also refer all patients to the public hospital.

Miller's motion was to be considered at the next monthly meeting of the hospital committee, that is, early in August. However, the annual general meeting of the hospital took place before then, on July 25. At this annual meeting, the largest for many years, elections to the committee were to be held, and tensions mounted as the agenda proceeded towards them. First there was the president's report, then the medical officer's. Both were positive. As medical officer, Dr. Little indicated that the hospital had had a good year medically. There had been 123 indoor and 32 outdoor patients. Ten deaths had occurred, including those of four patients whose ages ranged from sixty-seven to eighty-seven. There had been 22 cases of typhoid, with one death, and this marked a decrease over previous years. Despite the large number of surgical cases, there had been no surgical deaths. In short, Dr. Little as chief surgeon was able to submit a very satisfactory report.

At last came the elections. President Mackenzie was re-elected unopposed, but for the position of committeemen there were ten candidates and five places. The aggressive Mr. Miller came sixth and so lost his seat. His motion calling for the termination of Dr. Little's appointment was now deemed to have lapsed. Dr. Little must have breathed a sigh of relief and went to the August meeting of the committee believing that he was relatively safe. If so, he reckoned without Miller and his friends. In what seems like an obvious piece of petty collusion, the man who had just been elected as the fifth member of the committee resigned, and the president immediately appointed in his place the next in order of voting, none other than the outspoken Mr. Miller. The president also ruled that Miller's motion could be readmitted without notice.

The motion, reworded so that it became more evidently an attack on Dr. Little than a matter of principle, called for the termination of the medical officer's appointment at the end of three months (that is, October 30), sought fresh applications, and offered a salary of £150. That was an increase of £50 and was intended to compensate for any loss of income caused by the medical officer's being barred from any connection with a private hospital. Miller denied that the motion was a hostile one. He made a long speech about the reputation of the hospital, claiming that all members of the committee had heard complaints or, as he put it, "been twitted about the way in which things had been moving of late." He said it was known that Dr. Little preferred to have patients treated in a private hospital and referred to a case — Jewitt? — where the patient was taken away from the local hospital. Although Miller claimed that his resolution was not intended to cast a reflection on the medical officer, he was sure that subscribers would withdraw their support from the public hospital unless changes were made. He did concede that the resolution would not prevent Dr. Little from reapplying.

Dr. Little objected that the motion had been "sprung" on the committee, while his friends pointed out that the people were not in sympathy with Miller since they had failed to elect him. However, President Mackenzie overruled the objections, permitting the motion to go forward. The discussion, obviously heated, also dealt with the medical officer's salary, which one speaker claimed was the lowest in the district. Under the circumstances, it had been necessary for the doctor to supplement his income, not only through private practice, but also with an interest in a private hospital. It was noted that Dr. Little had made a "voluntary offer to retrench himself" when the hospital had been in financial difficulties. All this was recognized, but Miller and others thought that reforms must be made to put the hospital on a sound basis.

Dr. Little, obviously embattled and angry, said he did not know of any case where the hospital had been robbed. He said, "If there is a complaint, let it be in black and white. I would like any man to prove that I ever *robbed* the hospital of one patient. I have considered the hospital always. I am not going to attend wealthy patients for nothing."

After a good deal of discussion, during which it was again repeated that no slur upon Dr. Little was intended and the new salary was raised to £175 per annum, Miller's motion was put. It was a close thing, but it was carried. Dr. Little's appointment as medical officer of the Warracknabeal Hospital was to be terminated.

At the next monthly meeting of the committee, a new rule dealing with the appointment of the medical officer was accepted. This stipulated that the appointee "shall not have any interest in a Private Hospital" and required that any patient who made "the authorized declaration specified on the hospital admission form" must be recommended for treatment at the public hospital. Committeeman Miller did not think these requirements were sufficiently stringent, but ultimately accepted them. It was then decided that advertisements should be placed in the Melbourne newspapers. Thus, on September 4, 1901, the following notice appeared in *The Age* and *The Argus:*

> *Warracknabeal District Hospital*
> Applications are hereby called for the position of Medical Officer of the above institution. Non-residential private practice allowed. Salary £175 per annum. Applications close 30th September. . . . Full particulars on application to W.M. Candy, Sec.

In the scant two weeks allowed, four applications were received. These were to be voted upon at the hospital committee meeting of October 2. Once again, there was a noticeably large attendance at this meeting since the appointment of the medical officer was important enough in itself, but spice was added by the open quarrel between Dr. Little and Mr. Miller. When the votes were counted the final result was Dr. Ross — 10; Dr. Little — 7; Informal — 2. Dr. Ross was then declared medical officer-elect, to assume full duties on November 1, 1901. The matter seemed clearly settled: William C. Little had indeed lost his job as medical officer.

○ ○ ○

In the aftermath of the election, a committee member raised what seemed to be a merely academic question: "If Dr. Ross does not take up this position, will Dr. Little get the appointment because he is second in the voting?" He pointed out that this was the customary procedure of the committee and that it had been used recently with the appointment of both the new matron and two probationer nurses — not to mention Mr. Miller's appointment to the committee.

Mr. Miller quickly responded that this method did not apply to the medical officer. Another member commented that "the committee cannot prevent Dr. Little from applying, but they seem determined that he will not have the appointment." When the president was called upon for a ruling, he said that the meeting should decide. Thus a supportive motion was moved and seconded that "Dr. Little being the next highest in the poll, be selected in the case of Dr. Ross failing to accept." However, an amendment from the other camp called for fresh applications in the event that Dr. Ross withdrew. One argument given for this was that if Dr. Little were automatically reappointed, the issue of private hospitals would not have been properly addressed. The vote was then taken on the amendment. It was dead even, 9 — 9. All heads turned to President Mackenzie, who now had to cast his vote. His vote with the "ayes" was virtually a vote against Dr. Little. Thus it was determined that in the unlikely event of Dr. Ross not taking up his appointment, fresh applications for a medical officer would be sought.

It really did seem as if a faction of the committeemen was hostile to Dr. Little. What the reason might have been is impossible to determine. Small voluntary organizations in country towns can be as trenchantly political as major professional institutions in capital cities. The hostility of the participants is sometimes in inverse proportion to the goodness of their espoused cause, be it hospital or Red Cross or Benevolent Society. For a start, there is usually a clear division between town and country. Then there are old scores to settle and personal irritations to work off, all in addition to matters of high principle that are sometimes championed for the pettiest of reasons.

Committeeman Miller certainly led the attack against William Little, but whether for noble or base reasons is not clear. He seems to have been an outspoken and difficult person. For example, when it was moved that the committee compensate two nurses for the extra duties and responsibilities they willingly undertook in the extended absence of a matron, it was Miller who objected on the time-worn, sanctimonious grounds that "it would create an unfortunate precedent." It is easier to give the benefit of the doubt to President Mackenzie but he, too, was quite obviously no friend of W.C.L.'s. Other committeemen, however, did support him, and one even moved a motion to rescind the vote just taken. He recalled once again how Dr. Little had "been a good friend to the hospital when it had been in straitened circumstances." Such support must have been heartening, but all this discussion surely seemed an unnecessary expenditure of energy for, without doubt, Dr. Ross would take up the position for which he had so recently applied. However, such a conclusion would ignore the dynamics of life in small country towns and the esteem in which a country doctor may be held.

Dr. Ross was the medico in Dimboola, a town not far from Warracknabeal. On October 22, the Dimboola *Banner* reported that two delegations — the first of fifty men, the second of fifty women — had called upon

Dr. Ross to tell him they were pleased that he had won the job in Warracknabeal, but pleading with him to stay in Dimboola. Dr. Ross, who was taken by surprise, asked for time to reconsider. In the end, he sent a telegram to Warracknabeal declining the position of medical officer at the hospital. What had seemed a purely hypothetical question had now become a reality, and what a muddle it made! Dr. Little's tenure as medical officer expired on October 30th, and unless the motion that prevented him from automatically taking the position was rescinded, he was out and there would be no surgeon at the Warracknabeal Hospital.

The bemused committee partly solved the problem by refusing to accept Dr. Ross's resignation until December 1. Dr. Ross did not want to come from Dimboola to Warracknabeal to be medical officer for only one month, so he found a substitute for himself, appointing a Dr. Chapman as *locum tenens*. Dr. Little and his friends were furious that a man who had never actually been the medical officer should have the power to appoint to the position. The president of the hospital committee opined that it was not only Dr. Ross's right, but his responsibility to do that. The committee then called for new applications. Dr. Little did not reapply. This time, when the votes were counted, Dr. J.R. Lee, an honours graduate from Melbourne who had been practising in Omeo in the Gippsland area for three years, easily won. He was scheduled to take up his appointment on the first day of December.

Meanwhile, Dr. Ross's *locum,* Dr. Chapman, was still supposed to serve as medical officer during November. However, he left town without warning and without notifying Dr. Ross. The muddle at the hospital was getting worse. Dr. Ross tried to get Dr. Naylor of Minyip to act as M.O. for the month, but that gentleman wired that "he was strictly neutral" and wanted to stay out of the mess. The doctor from Hopetoun was of the same mind. Finally, Dr. Theed, an honorary medical officer at Warracknabeal, agreed to be acting medical officer. Before the month was little more than half over, Dr. Theed had cause to regret that decision, for on November 18th, the hospital was faced with its second medical scandal of 1901.

○　○　○

Around 5 p.m. on November 18th, Thomas Logan, a resident of the village of Hopetoun, was brought to acting Medical Officer Theed. He had a severe abdominal complaint, and Dr. Theed sent a man to the president of the hospital committee to acquire an order of admission, which was duly issued. Theed determined that the case was serious, that surgery would be needed and, at 6:30 p.m. wired to Dr. Ross, who was technically still the medical officer and surgeon of the hospital: "Patient requiring chloroform. Urgent. Come at once." Dr. Ross wired back from Dimboola: "Ask Dr. Little give chloroform. Reply paid."

This response was received after 8 p.m., when the telegraph office closed.

Meanwhile, nothing had been done for the patient. He was kept waiting still longer as Theed conferred with the hospital committee. The president asked the acting M.O. to ask Dr. Little to participate in the operation as Dr. Ross had suggested. Dr. Theed had already told the hospital committee that he "personally would not touch the patient on any consideration for fear of conveying blood poisoning to his private patients," but he did ask Dr. Little to perform the operation. Dr. Little, after all the politicking that had been going on, "declined to recognize Dr. Ross in the matter," but would have performed the operation on the written authorization of the hospital committee. Dr. Theed confidently arranged for a cab to stand by to pick up Dr. Little to take him to the hospital and reported this to the committee.

Given the history of Dr. Little's recent relationship with the hospital, together with the fact that Dr. Theed held the opinion that it was "rather too late" and "that there was hardly a shadow of hope that the patient would recover," Little's request for formal authorization was quite professional and eminently reasonable. It should not have added to the delay. However, the hospital committee did not take advantage of his willingness to serve — though he had so recently been their house surgeon. Instead, they told Theed to wire back to Dr. Ross. By this time of night, the telegram office was firmly closed, and Dr. Theed refused to "tramp off to the railway station to send a wire from there." The house committee then, at 11 p.m., chose to rouse the stationmaster and, "so as to keep faith with Dr. Ross," wired him to come the following morning.

It was now very late and dark; everyone was tired and agitated; further action that day was impossible. Dr. Theed cancelled the cab and, let us hope, Dr. Little was informed that his services would not be required. Dr. Ross arrived from Dimboola the next day, claiming he had not realized how serious the situation was, and proceeded to operate. Poor Thomas Logan finally had his surgery. He seemed to come through it satisfactorily, but a day or two later he suffered a severe haemorrhage and, on December 9, he died. The unfortunate fellow would probably have died anyway, but his case was certainly not improved by the delays.

These seemed to have been the unhappy result of the politics of the hospital committee and its unwillingness to call upon Dr. Little. It looked as though the committee of laymen had put a personal vendetta above the welfare of a patient. Dr. Theed said publicly that Dr. Little had made it clear he was available. Theed went further. He said that the committee should have formally asked Dr. Little and that "in the opinion of most people it would have been the proper and most humane course to have pursued." Letters in local papers supported that view. They ran strongly in Dr. Little's favour and decried "the plot to dispense with his services." Dr. Little did not stand idly by in the aftermath of the Logan case. On the day after Logan's death, Dr. Little lodged with the police a formal demand that a full inquiry be made. However, the coroner ruled that there was no need for an investigation. Nothing more could be done, so the burial of Logan proceeded.

The case was not entirely closed. Dr. Ross, who found himself embroiled in an unexpected furore, fired Dr. Theed as his *locum*. He then had more trouble than ever trying to find a replacement. Even the honorary medical officers resigned from the Warracknabeal Hospital. The townspeople, in their letters to *The Northern Argus,* also called for the resignation of the hospital committee. Warracknabeal must have been in an uproar, split by a great public controversy. This began to subside after Dr. John Lee took over as medical officer in December. Thus the year ended with a weary and harassed Dr. W.C. Ross going off on his "lengthy holiday," while a disillusioned and disappointed Dr. W.C. Little severed forever his official ties with the Warracknabeal Hospital.

The man who had been willing to attempt the difficult operation that the acting medical officer would not touch was not the man to leave the district with his head down. Dr. Little stayed in Warracknabeal and continued to serve the community as Public Vaccinator and District Health Officer. The private hospital, which had been such an integral part of the row with the public hospital committeemen, then became the central focus of his professional life. William Little was not unscathed, but he had managed to survive the pitfalls of 1901 and the storm of hospital politics.

o   o   o

About a decade before all this hassle with the Warracknabeal Hospital began, Billy Little had written to Grace Ritchie, "If I were rich, I would ask you to take a trip around the world with me" (July 6, 1890). About a decade after the big to-do with Committeeman Miller *et al.*, Dr. Little's dream of a global tour was partly fulfilled. Sure enough, he made his trip

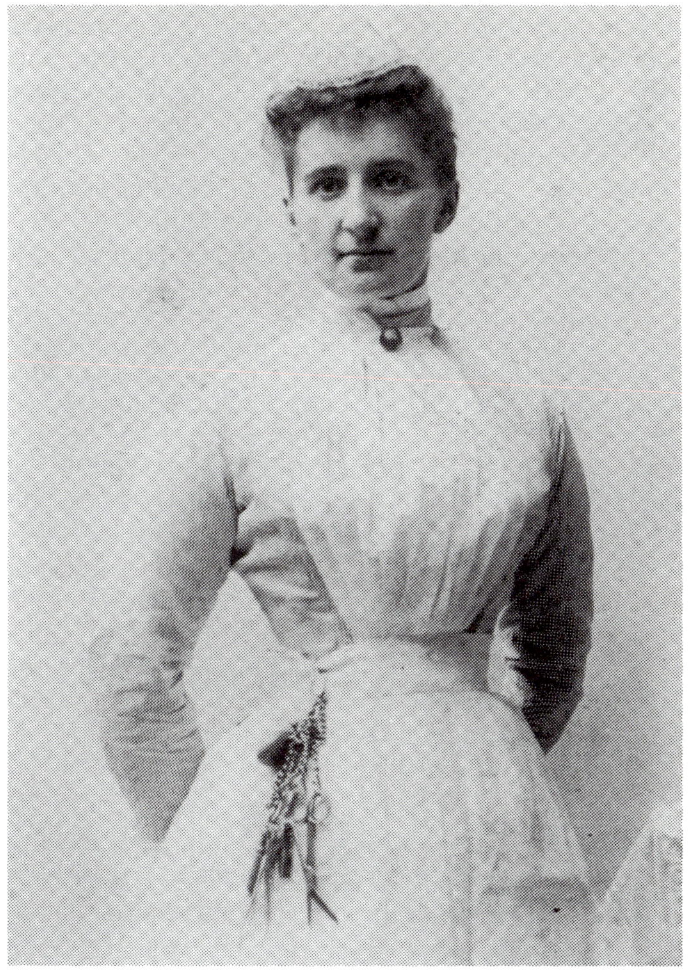

Nurse Jenny Gaff

around the world, and he even visited some of his old haunts in Scotland and Canada, though he did so, not with Grace Ritchie, but in the company of Nurse Jenny Gaff.

Janet (Jenny) Muir Steel was born in Scotland in 1860, the same year as William Little. She grew up in "the old country," trained as a nurse in Glasgow, married a man called Daniel Gaff, and had one son, Dan junior. Dan Gaff senior is a man of mystery. Glimpses of him from members of the Steel family suggest variously that he was rich, very old, and went to the altar in a wheelchair, or that he was a charming "ne'er-do-well" who squandered his money, or that he was a wastrel who abandoned his wife and child in order to seek his fortune in North America. There is no substantiation for any of these versions of Dan Gaff, but it is known from shipping lists that he did not accompany his wife and son when they, together with other members of the Steel family — father, mother, and sisters Helen and Marion — migrated to Australia in 1891–92. According to written records left by Marion Steel, Nurse Jenny Gaff met Dr. William C. Little when he was on a visit to Melbourne in 1892. She was then working as a private nurse at Camperdown, and he was on the look-out for well-trained staff for the new Warracknabeal public hospital.

W.C.L., who did not always have a high opinion of nurses (July 6, 1890; February 18, 1891), was impressed by Jenny Gaff and he was successful in recruiting her. She began work at the Warracknabeal Hospital before the year was out. In a letter to Grace Ritchie (June 8, 1893), W.C.L. commented on a photograph he had enclosed: "That nurse standing is the best trained nurse I have met in my medical experience." It is more than likely that this otherwise unidentified woman was Jenny Gaff, for it was she with whom he chose to work in his private hospital. From 1896, she was technically the lessor of Massawippi, then she bought the building in 1901, and he bought it from her the following year — shortly after his *contretemps* with the public hospital. Jenny Gaff remained on the municipal records as the occupier of the premises until 1908, and there are frequent references in the Warracknabeal newspapers during this period to "Nurse Gaff's Hospital."

The memories of Jenny Gaff within the Steel family are of sun and shadow. On the one hand there seems to be no doubt that she was a strong, vital person. Her photograph suggests as much. Her nephew, Archibald Steel, remembers her in later life as a woman of striking appearance, with a good figure and stately carriage, generally wearing an imposing string of amber beads. He recalls that she was kind, had a sense of humour and that he preferred her to his other aunts, her sisters Marion and Helen. Yet on the other hand, these sisters spoke of Jenny with a sort of hush and children were hastily banished from the room if her personal affairs were being discussed. Marion Steel wrote some introductory notes to Jenny's diaries in which she enigmatically promised, "Some day I may tell you a few items (PRIVATE)" — but she never did. Those secrets about Jenny went to the grave with members of her generation.

In Warracknabeal, as on the boat to Australia, Jenny was called "Miss Gaff" or "Nurse Gaff," so she was presumed to be unmarried. Her son stayed with the Steel family in Melbourne, thus his existence was not generally known. There is nothing so unusual or clandestine about all this, but it does tend to make Jenny's status rather nebulous, places a small skeleton in her closet, makes her the subject of whispers. Still, as far as Billy Little was concerned, she was a real and stalwart presence and an increasingly important part of his life in Warracknabeal.

Somewhere about the time that Massawippi was relinquished, Dr. Little's health began to fail. Over the years, he had had a number of serious bouts of illness and traces of these appear in the correspondence with Grace Ritchie. For example, the last letter (March 16, 1894) clearly indicated he had been so sick with typhoid that "he was so thin you could read a newspaper through him" and "almost tie a knot in his legs." Although he described himself as having recovered and grown "succulent," his once robust constitution was undermined. He suffered a recurrence of typhoid, reportedly when he "foolishly stroked his moustache while attending a typhoid patient."[11] Steel family legend has it that Jenny pulled him through when he was very ill and all hope was gone. She did it more with bravado than medicine: she smashed a bottle of champagne on his iron bed, poured it down his throat and watched the happy results!

Not surprisingly, that "cure" was not long-lasting, but Dr. Little was later able to prescribe for himself a world tour — "home" to Scotland, home to Canada, then home to Australia. If the trip to Ceylon so many years ago had "brought back his color, rejuvenated his nerves and given him a new lease on life," then long ocean voyages could do the same again. After all, he was only fifty years old. Dr. R.A. Stirling, a long-time colleague and friend who practised in Melbourne and whom Dr. Little consulted about his own health, consented to his taking the trip on the condition that W.C.L. did not travel alone. The obvious person to accompany him was Nurse Gaff. She was professionally trained and would be able to look after him if he were really ill on the voyage.

William Little's relationship to Jenny Gaff was a subject of much speculation and gossip in Warracknabeal. One old-timer in that town forthrightly asserted that "she had been his matron and his mistress"[12] for many years. That is one interpretation. Members of the Steel family believed that Dr. Little fell in love with Jenny and wanted to marry her; that they tried without success to find Dan Gaff because she was not free to marry if he were still alive; that the trip abroad was an effort to locate him; that, though Dan Gaff had deserted his wife many years before and the marriage could therefore be legally dissolved, "Dr. Little had strong views on marrying a divorced woman."[13] As for Jenny, "she made a perfect god of the man."[14] Throughout her diary, all references to Billy Little are to "The Doctor" or to "H.R.H." — His Royal Highness.

Dr. Little was fully aware of the power of rumors: ". . . people will talk and this place is the essence of Gossip. Mrs. Grundy flourishes here like a big sun flower" (February 16, 1890). Yet somehow, the idea of his not wanting to marry Nurse Gaff because she was a married woman does not ring true. Even given that divorce was a disgrace in the early years of the twentieth century, surely a professional man in a small country town would risk more opprobrium for openly having a mistress, a doctor for cohabiting with the matron of his hospital, than for having a wife who happened to have been married before. Dr. Little indicated several times in his letters that he was sensitive to hierarchy, to social/professional distance, so was it a question of doctor/nurse status? Or was it for love of Grace Ritchie that Billy Little chose not to marry the good, kind, competent woman who was virtually his partner in practice and who all but worshipped him? Or did she decline his offer? Or was there another reason?

○　○　○

On Friday, March 4, 1910, Dr. William C. Little, accompanied by Nurse Janet M.S. Gaff, sailed eastward out of Sydney harbour, bound for Britain via New Zealand, Cape Horn, and the stormy Atlantic. They did not share a cabin. Jenny recorded in her diary that "H.R.H.'s cabin companion is a Navy Lieutenant" who was amusing and who played golf. She noted icebergs, whales, sailing ships at sea, and many of the curiosities of life in foreign ports — the hotel in Montevideo overcharged for lunch, the harbour in Rio de Janeiro was grander than Sydney's, the money changers carefully "rang their gold" before they accepted it, prices were four times higher than in Melbourne. Arriving in London two days before the death of King Edward VII, they experienced the heart of Empire in royal mourning, witnessed the funeral and "did" the mandatory tourist places. W.C.L. kept up the pace. Then on to Ireland, where they decided that to kiss the Blarney Stone was too dangerous, but they braved the Devil's Causeway, observed baby donkeys from train windows, and noted the costs of grand new buildings. Then back to England for more sightseeing, also an encounter with Susan Little, W.C.L.'s youngest sister, who was visiting Britain. The strain of all this began to tell. Nurse Gaff noted: "H.R.H. far from well," so she spent "a whole day in Doctor's room mending." In June they were off again, this time to Norway, sailing up the fjords, utterly impressed with the beauty and magnificence of it all. "H.R.H.," for some reason, would "not permit" Kristiansund to be visited. His ruling was not questioned. They saw a spectacular midnight sun, "very low and making a golden glow across the water," visited Hamerfest, the most northerly town in Europe, came south to tour the Lofoten Islands, bought some enamelled buttons in Trondheim, and at Molde, "Doctor feels much better for being here. Saturday rested, went for a little walk. Doctor bought me a lovely necklace of filigree."

So they progressed. By late July, they found themselves in Scotland, where they alternated between "quiet times," seeing relatives, and shopping. (She bought the amber beads in Aberdeen and he bought her "a pretty brooche" in Inverness.) Some days "Doctor rested." On September 14, they went to Ecclefechan, visited four graveyards, found the tombstone of Doctor's great-great-grandmother, saw the spot where Robert the Bruce slew the Red Comyn. London again. Paris. Genoa. Pisa. Rome — "the Forum is too magnificent for words." Naples — "H.R.H. very tired so rested all afternoon." Capri — "H.R.H. taken round Pompeii in a chair." Rome again and, just when all seemed to be going well, a dramatic, anguished entry:

> October 26 — What a terrible time I've had since the 15th. Doctor got ptomaine poisoning and has been dreadfully ill. So sick for four days and then delusions for four days. Have the best doctor in Florence, Professor Giglioli, and now a masseur. I've been night and day and the anxiety has been awful. Away by myself and only my own self. The four days' delirium was awful. Night and day picking up things that weren't there. Oh! It was so pitiful to see such a fine man in such a terrible state. These last three days, gentle, steady progress has been made, but another setback last night as the massage had been too severe and caused great pain and doctor had no sleep. Oh how I wish I could get him better. This October 26th I feel nervous and broken down for want of rest.

Poor Jenny Gaff! What a terrible responsibility she had — so far from home, unable to speak the languages of Europe, her companion/employer so startlingly ill. No wonder she felt "broken down." Relentlessly, their tour continued.

Venice. Milan. Lucerne — luxurious rooms at l'Hotel du Lac. Back to London. Booked passage to Canada. "Doctor" bought Jenny "the loveliest watch" at Mappin and Webbs for £10. Sailed on the *Hisperion.* The food was good, but "H.R.H. pretty sick all the time." Arrived in Halifax, Nova Scotia, the week before Christmas, 1910, and spent the holidays with his sister, Elizabeth Little Chase, and her family. Jenny noted: "Have spent a most enjoyable eight days at this most hospitable home. Everyone is so kind and I'm made to feel as one of the family." In Nova Scotia, with W.C.L.'s

Left at 10 am. 29th reached ~~Otta~~
Ottawa 1 p.m. ~~stayed~~ at Russel Hotel
visited Parliament building which are
very fine & magnificent. In ——
had a fine sleigh drive by the frozen
river & canals fine. Left next morning
30th at 11 am. Ottawa & d. had to change
~~trains~~ at Smith's Falls. Fearfully cold.
Montreal train & our late came in both
engine coated with ice. Were glad to
stay in Ottawa rain till ——. Came in
Ottawa & whole country under snow.
Dined on car & afternoon tea reached
Toronto about 9 p.m. being about 2 hours
late. Miss ~~Little~~ met us. Mr. & Mrs. ——
glad to see J. Went for sleigh drive
next day the 31st. So say good bit of city
Jan 1st went to church at night. ——
Also Jan 5th had another fine sleigh
ride. J. got ill 11th great abscess
broke in bowel. Was very ill has been
in bed now for over 2 weeks but is
able to be up now the 28th. I've
been about the city a lot so have

A page from Jenny Gaff's diary

sister and her daughters, Lillian and Margaret, they "had some fine drives to quaint towns which somehow conveyed the impression of up-country Australia."

On they went, through New Brunswick by train and thence to Montreal in late January. What were William Little's feelings as he returned to this city where he had spent that happy time more than two decades before? Had he forgotten Grace Ritchie? Did she still tug at his heart? Did he try to see her? Did he, indeed, meet her? Jenny Gaff's diary, the only known record of this visit, reads simply:

> Reached Montreal 10.00 in the morning. Stayed at Windsor Hotel. Montreal deep in snow. Went sleighing. Saw grain elevators and river all frozen over. It's a great sight. Montreal is a very fine city. Saw McGill University and all the splendid colleges. Booked at C.P. for Australia via *Zealandia* to sail Vancouver.

No mention of people, no note of W.C.L.'s physical condition. But there was much about the latter during their two weeks in Toronto, where William Little saw his parents for the first time in so very long. It was also to be the last time he would be with them. On January 8th, "Doctor got ill and a great abscess broke into his bowel." He stayed in bed for two weeks while Jenny explored Toronto with his sister Susan and friends. She thought it, too, was "a very fine city," but considered the "shops on the whole inferior to Melbourne's." On February 8th, another hydatid cyst burst, but two days later, W.C.L. was able to do a little visiting in Toronto. Then they were back on the train, heading west across the prairies, where Jenny Gaff saw with her Australian eyes, "Deep snow for hundreds of miles, not one tree, a continuous plain, reminding one of the country from Murtoa to Warracknabeal." Banff, the Rockies, the Selkirks drew forth much awestruck, admiring description. Vancouver, too. At last the voyage home, during which she read *The Last Days of Pompeii* to him but, as they approached Australia's shores, it must have been obvious that this grand and expensive tour had not achieved its goal of "putting the color back into his cheeks." She recorded the sad fact that "Doctor has been really ill for two days, so I have not been out of the cabin." On Sunday, February 26, they reached Sydney and took the overnight train back to Melbourne. So much for the world tour.

○　○　○

The *Warracknabeal Herald* greeted Dr. Little's return with warmth and respect, but, before many months were out, another local paper, the *Dunmunkle Standard* of Murtoa, announced a different kind of trip. In its issue of September 8, 1911, the *Standard* included the following item:

> At the request of Dr. W.C. Little, whose health has been unsatisfactory for some time, his medical advisor, Dr. Stirling, paid a visit to Warracknabeal on Monday, travelling by special train and returning to Melbourne the same day.

The chartering of a special train made a great impression in the district, but the outcome of the expedition was not successful. William C. Little's health continued to deteriorate. Stories circulated about his bizarre behaviour, rumour had it that he was drinking or taking drugs. Yet another special train was ordered. This one for Dr. Little and Nurse Gaff, to take them to Melbourne, where he was admitted to Pine Grove, a private hospital in Lennox Street, Richmond. It was there that William Little died on October 6, 1911. His old friend, Dr. R. Stirling, who was in attendance, attributed the cause of death to acute pneumonia. It was a final blessed release from those many months of suffering. The day after his death, Dr. Little was buried in Boroondarra Cemetery, Melbourne.

○ ○ ○

In his will, made after twenty-one years in Victoria, William C. Little remembered his Canadian roots, bequeathing something to all members of his immediate family. A legacy of £1,000 went to each of his six sisters (or, since Dr. Isabel had died of typhoid in Canton, to her daughter), while a very generous £3,000 was left to his brother James of Melbourne. His parents were given the rights to the house where they lived, as well as income from other property in Toronto. (W.C.L. had obviously purchased all this property to help his father out of financial difficulties, perhaps those "little troubles" mentioned in the last part of the last letter to Grace Ritchie.) For Grace Ritchie-England there was nothing in William Little's will, but for Janet Muir Steel Gaff there was the sum of £3,000, a sizable amount that gave her a degree of independence for the rest of her life. It enabled her to go abroad again, especially after the First World War. (During the war, she travelled widely under less than agreeable circumstances as a nurse on a hospital ship.) Her son, Dan Gaff, was not forgotten in Dr. Little's will. He received £50, plus the doctor's piano. Other small bequests included £50 to a housekeeper, £100 to the Warracknabeal Presbyterian Church, and £50 to the Warracknabeal Hospital. William C. Little had worked hard, amassed a respectable estate, and distributed it even-handedly. Like many an immigrant, he had chosen to remember the people in the land of his birth as well as those in the country of his adoption.

Long after his death, Dr. Little was warmly remembered in Warracknabeal and the surrounding district. While several informants spoke of his "bizarre behaviour," his "little weakness," and suspected heavy drinking towards the end, their recollections or inherited impressions of him were very positive. The town's historian formally recorded his interest in the area, noting how, among other things, improved public health was attributed to his recommendation that trees be planted along the Yarriambiac Creek. [14] The sugar gums that were planted around Warracknabeal did help reduce typhoid. Even if the cause was not that the foliage improved "the air's vital quality" as Dr. Little predicted, but that the roots absorbed the stagnant pools of water that allowed typhoid-bearing mosquitos to breed, the prescription worked and Dr. Little was duly given credit. He also earned more personal approval through his concern for his patients so that, more than seventy years later, there were still those in Warracknabeal who remembered his name with affection. He had become the stuff of family legend.

There is, for example, a story in the Fletcher family of a young girl who got her thumb all but cut off when it was caught in an overturned cart. She was rushed bleeding and screaming to Dr. Little's surgery, where the good doctor, faced with a terrified child and a difficult job of stitching, shrewdly said, "This won't take long to chop off!" To which the child spunkily replied, as he had known she would, "No you don't!" and then she willingly kept still while he sewed the severed member back on. She proudly kept that thumb until she died at ninety. Other anecdotes still circulate in Warracknabeal concerning how Dr. Little saved someone's mother's life, or how he would never give up on a case, or how he was willing to try new or even radical procedures if all else had failed.

Billy Little, the farmer's son from Ontario, never expected to become famous or to be the subject of anecdote in the Antipodes. Neither did he intend to spend his entire professional life in far-off Australia; nor, for that matter, did he anticipate having his personal letters to Grace Ritchie published almost a century later. He might have been startled or even embarrassed by this, but he would have immensely enjoyed his claim to local fame in Warracknabeal and, let us hope, would have been happy enough to share his experiences with other people in Canada and Australia. "Good heavings!" he might say, or "Great United States!" — in surprise and amusement at such an unlikely turn of events.

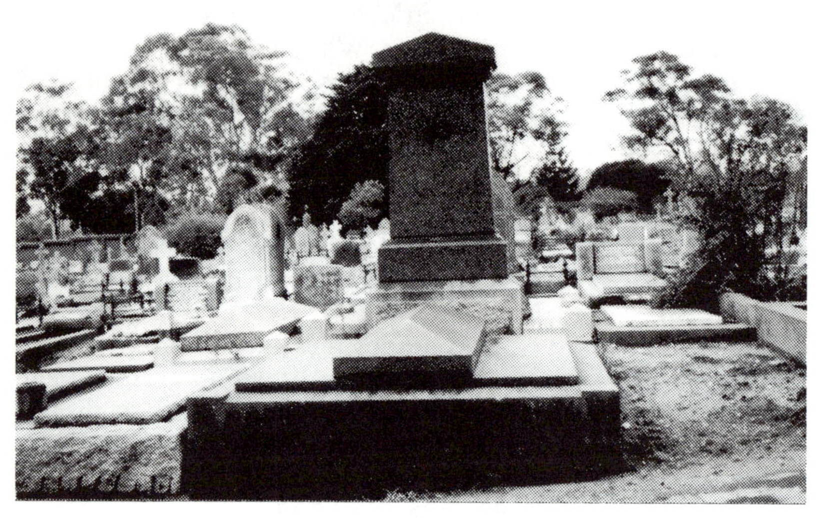

Boroondara Cemetery, Melbourne
The flat grave in the foreground
bears the inscription:

In Memory Of
WILLIAM CLOW LITTLE, M.D.
BELOVED SON OF
ROBERT AND SUSANNAH LITTLE, CANADA
BORN 1ST APRIL 1860,
DIED IN MELBOURNE 6TH OCTOBER 1911
UNTIL THE DAY BREAKS AND THE SHADOWS FALL AWAY

PART V

All Stones Turned?

All Stones Turned?

There, Reviewer B! Are you surprised at how much has been uncovered about William Little, the unknown Canadian physician? Are you satisfied that this project has proved to be an opportunity to discover both the writer and the recipient of the letters, to acknowledge both William Little and Grace Ritchie? Have your doubts dissolved?

If you have read this far, you must have realized that the pursuit of Billy Little required a second visit to Australia. That trip took place during my sabbatic leave in 1985–86 and was as enjoyable and as filled with fortunate circumstances as the previous one. The renewed inquiry in Australia aroused interest from more people, produced additional information, brought new insights and shed light on at least two important pieces of the puzzle — the diaries of Jenny Gaff and the events of 1901.

Nurse Gaff's diaries were willingly made available to me by Mrs. Gwen Steel of Frankston, Victoria — not only the diaries themselves, but also a typescript of part of them, plus a sheaf of correspondence gathered when Mrs. Steel was working on "The Steel Family History." This material contained some additional fragments, recollections from family members and Warracknabeal residents who had known both Jenny Gaff and Billy Little. Mr. Archibald Steel, the nephew of Jenny Gaff, was able to recall his aunt with considerable clarity. Thus, altogether, I was lucky enough to encounter a descendant of Grace Ritchie (in the person of Mrs. Esther England Cushing), Billy Little (in the person of Dr. Lillian Chase), and Jenny Gaff (in the person of Mr. Archie Steel). Those human contacts, along with the primary sources, greatly enriched my quest.

Of course, not everything was smooth sailing. My arrival in Melbourne happened to coincide with the first full-scale closing of the Victorian State Library (for stocktaking) in more than a hundred years. My perusal of the Warracknabeal newspapers was seriously delayed. Yet this initial bad luck was more offset by the fact that when I got to the papers I found that there had been some very assiduous reporters attending the meetings of the hospital committee throughout 1901, and they had left a lot of material for me to gather. Meanwhile, there were many other sources to explore.

The obvious, if unessential matter of W.C.L.'s birthday had not yielded to inquiries at the obvious places for, curiously, all the educational institutions where he had been registered and which would have been expected to have noted his date of birth either had no records at all or held incomplete data on him. The shipping lists were suggested as a possible way to identify the elusive "crazy day" — but they revealed only age, not date of birth. Still the letter Billy Little wrote in mid-March 1894, mentioning his forthcoming birthday strongly supported April 1, and, at last, records at Booroondara General Cemetery confirmed that theory.

The pursuit continued. Probate records in Melbourne led to archives in Laverton, Victoria, and a great tome with a copy of W.C.L.'s will. A seminar dealing with this project arranged by Professor Richard Selleck at Monash University proved to be surprisingly lively when some members of the audience — "Ding" Dyason, Doug and Evie McColl, Joan Utber, John Schubert, and Gwen Steel — found that they were part of the content. Even an illness turned out to have fortunate side effects, for it introduced me to Dr. Frank Forster, one of Australia's most distinguished historians of medicine, and he referred me to Ms. Ann Tovell, the well-informed and helpful archivist of the Australian Medical Association . . . . And so it went.

For all that, one old question remained unanswered: "What about the cattle at Windsor Castle?" Neither Guelph, Ottawa, nor a direct inquiry to Windsor Castle archives revealed anything further about W.C.L.'s involvement in the purchasing trip of 1884. There seemed to be no other stones to turn on this relatively trivial item and the major questions had been addressed satisfactorily. Did that mean, therefore, that the investigation into the life and times of Billy Little was at an end?

When can a researcher be absolutely certain that no stone has been left unturned, that all the significant facts are in so that wise selections can be made from them, so that the tale can unfold fully and interpretations be presented with minimal distortion? How far afield must the inquiry go? The answers to these questions are relative and must vary according to circumstances but, if it is permissible to be dogmatic about anything, it would be to say that the last word is never in and that there will always be room for revision (and revisionism) in the writing of history. Still, each project must come to an end some time. When this is to be will be determined basically by the integrity and judgment of the researcher, often in the face of extrinsic pressures such as institutional requirements, publishers' deadlines, and other practicalities. The researcher must decide when the law of diminishing returns will take over, when tackling one more vague lead would not be worth the time and effort needed.

The researcher also has to grapple with the problem of what known material to exclude. In the case of Billy Little, this writer had to restrain herself from exploring in greater detail the apparent, if superficial, similarity between two medical doctors in nineteenth-century Victoria, "my" Dr. William C. Little and the Dr. Richard Mahony of Henry Handel Richardson's great Australian novel. The more I learned about Billy Little, the more I could see common themes — the country, the sense of distance, the alienation of the immigrant, marriage, and money. On reflection, I concluded that literary excursions really did not fit in *Dear Grace* and should be left for another occasion.

Once these problems of scope have been dealt with, there are others of organization and style. How many footnotes are needed? How intrusive will it be to have all sources fully noted and explanations freely offered? In the case of Billy Little's letters, will there be some things that Canadian readers might not understand about Australia, and Australians about Canada? How much extra does the historian pack into footnotes, those delicious little tidbits that could not properly be fitted into the text but that were too good to throw away and might never be of any real use except, perhaps, as answers to some rarified "Trivial Pursuit"? The treatment of technicalities of this kind may be largely dictated by space constraints, publishers' policies, and the like, but the writer still has to make the basic decision. If that means fewer rather than more notes, then the writer has to be sure that he or she has played fair with the reader in order that there is sufficient trust so that every statement does not need to be substantiated, every detail accounted for.

Then the writer might wonder how much will the reader bring to the book? When might explanations seem like condescension? How many questions can legitimately be left unanswered? How far should the writer stray beyond the data presented? Should he or she try to propose answers to motivational questions like "Why did Billy Little never marry?" "Why did he not return to Canada?" "Why did he stay in Warracknabeal?" From the information now available, such questions could only be answered hypothetically, not conclusively. Nevertheless, tentative responses could lead to some interesting and even unexpected possibilities. Is it feasible, for example, that all the above questions about Billy Little's motives could be answered by one startling hypothesis — namely, that Billy Little was the victim of syphilis?

An hypothesis of that kind would be impossible to prove but might be reasonable enough to explore. Supporting considerations might include:

• The fact that it would have been very easy for any young man to contract syphilis in the Victoria of the 1880s and '90s. Venereal disease was virtually unchecked and uncheckable. While it is likely that W.C.L. would not have contracted such a disease in Warracknabeal, he could certainly have done so in Melbourne, either when he first arrived or on later visits. He says "the very old devil takes possession of me sometimes" (August 3, 1890, and September 28, 1890) and that he needed to break out from the constraints of "being so precise, always looking and acting the Dr." (August 3, 1890). And again, "I know it is wrong, but then I love to do wrong things sometimes for the experience" (April 14, 1891). Any kind of sexual adventure he might have undertaken on those occasions would have carried a high risk of syphilis.

• If W.C.L. did contract such a disease he, as a medical man, would have been fully aware of his condition and that he "could not honourably marry." It is conceivable that this is the real reason why he did not wed Jenny Gaff. The propositions that Dan Gaff senior could not be found or that Jenny would have borne the taint of being a divorced woman seem flimsy excuses for a vigorous man not to marry a woman he respected and with whom he chose to spend a good deal of his time. Marriage would have stopped rather than added to gossip.

• The knowledge of his condition, with the associated embarrassment and shame, would also act as a deterrent against his going back to his family in Canada.

• The description of his final illness is consistent with the symptoms of the tertiary stages of syphilis, which can take from ten to twenty years to manifest themselves fully. The complaints recorded in Nurse Gaff's diary, namely hydatid cysts and ptomaine poisoning, do not account for the hallucinations and the severity of W.C.L.'s illness during the world tour: "Night and day picking up things that weren't there. Oh! It was so pitiful to see such a fine man in such a terrible state." The "bizarre behaviour" and apparent drunkeness noted by some Warracknabeal residents in his later days might also be attributed to the disease, as might the difficulties that required his being taken through Pompeii on a chair and having massage in Florence. "Acute pneumonia," the diagnosis made by Dr. Stirling on Dr. Little's death certificate, does not necessarily invalidate the syphilis hypothesis. Pneumonia or pulmonary failure may commonly be the culmination of illnesses conditioned by other causes.

The syphilis hypothesis is certainly not the preferred one to leave with the reader. However, once issues like this have been raised, considered, and judged to have some validity, does the researcher not have an obligation to present them, even at the risk of spoiling the image of the subject? If, indeed, William Little did suffer from this dread disease, would it not be expected that twentieth-century readers would sympathize rather than condemn? Would they not see new, darker, more tragic dimensions to his character, facets that would take nothing away from the ebullient young Canadian who set forth to make his fortune in Australia and who wrote such lively letters to his dear Grace?

Historical judgments always run a certain risk of "present-mindedness" or interpreting the past from the mind-set of the present, but this should not be confused with the showing of sympathetic understanding of the past. Indeed, the latter is one of the desirable outcomes of writing or reading history. Yet another risk the historian runs is the distorting effect of his or her broad theories or particular notions. In this case, did an initial resemblance noted between Dr. William C. Little and the fictional Dr. Richard Mahony contribute unduly to the syphilis hypothesis? More important, was this a strained or an unfair connection? Was there determinism at work in this project as well as systematic inquiry and serendipity? The answers to questions such as these may just raise still further questions, so that the pursuit of Billy Little may continue, not as a quest for information about that individual, but as an ongoing inquiry into the nature of doing history.

NOTES

PART II — BACKGROUNDS

1. *Historical Atlas of Simcoe County, Ontario,* H. Belden & Co., 1881, p.7.

2. Another graduate from the Barrie school was William Osler (1849–1919) who made major contributions to clinical medicine and medical education.

3. He says that it seemed to be his fate to go everywhere twice. He visited Ceylon again on his way to Australia in 1889. Ceylon twice, Britain twice — i.e., once for the livestock, once for medical studies?

4. The first Canadian woman to earn a medical degree was Emily Stowe. She got her M.D. in 1867 but had to go to New York for it. Her daughter, Augusta, became the first Canadian woman to receive the degree in Canada (Victoria College, Cobourg, 1883).

5. Adam Shortt Papers, Queen's University Archives.

6. Elizabeth Smith Shortt, *Historical Sketch of Medical Education of Women, Kingston, Canada,* Ottawa: Private Printing, 1916, p. 1.

7. Threats of migration were common in the early days of universities and were taken seriously. Mediaeval students used these as powerful weapons against professors or civic authorities that they did not like. Cambridge was originally a migration from Oxford.

8. Margaret Gillett, *We Walked Very Warily: A History of Women at McGill,* Montreal: Eden Press, 1981, p. 109.

9. R.A. Cage, ed., *The Scots Abroad: Labour, Capital, Enterprise, 1750-1914,* London: Croom Helm, 1985.

10. Walter Lindesay Richardson, quoted in Dorothy Green, "Walter Lindesay Richardson: The Man, the Portrait, the Artist," *Meanjin,* 1 (1970), 5.

11. "Australian Characteristics," *The Northern Argus,* September 3, 1891, p. 4.

12. Tuberculosis.

13. Susan Priestly, *Warracknabeal — A Wimmera Centenary,* Brisbane & Melbourne: Jacaranda Press, 1967, p. 26.

14. *The Northern Argus,* August 6, 1891, p. 2 — but Bruck gives the population in 1892 as 1,320, while in 1896 he cites 2,500.

15. Editorial, *The Northern Argus,* May 21, 1891, p. 2.

PART III — THE LETTERS, 1889–1894

1. Doctor of Medicine, Master of Surgery, Member of the College of Physicians and Surgeons of Ontario, Licentiate of the Royal College of Surgeons Edinburgh.

2. A transverse fracture of the radius just above the wrist.

3. A small textbook, *Obstetrics and Gynaecology,* which was considered by a reviewer in the *Queen's Medical Review* to be "very complete for its size and furnished to the students of his time a class-book always eagerly sought after by them." Dr. Kenneth W. Fenwick (1852–1896), Professor of Gynaecology and Obstetrics at the Royal College of Surgeons, Kingston, was the lecturer in Physiology who was so hostile to the pioneer women medical students — Elizabeth Smith, Alice McGillivray, et al. It seems ironic that Billy Little should mention him in this favourable manner to Grace.

   Dr. A.A. Travill has observed that Fenwick's attempt to destroy medical co-education was the only serious blemish on his career, pointing out in his "History of Medicine at Queen's" that Fenwick's "discourtesy to the lady students . . . does not seem to have been held against him for any considerable time because by the end of the decade 1880's he held the Chair of Surgery in the Kingston Women's Medical College." Fenwick published a paper that would certainly have pleased Grace — it was on "Women's Dress Reform" (*Queen's College Journal,* XVIII, 1889/90, 177–78). Furthermore, he was highly regarded as a teacher and was a favourite of the medical students. He died prematurely as a result of an infection in a small cut received on his hand while performing surgery. Gangrene developed, he refused to have his arm amputated and so he died. The Queen's community mourned him as "one more martyr . . . called to the rolls of medical heroes." That such a popular man should have been ringleader against those worthy female students illustrates the complexity and difficulty of women's acceptance into professional spheres. It would have been so much easier for Elizabeth Smith, Alice McGillivray and their colleagues to have had to contend with an unpopular, churlish opponent. "Nice" men who give lip service to feminist causes make very formidable enemies.

4. A small town 49 miles north-west of Montreal.

5. Harriette Walker and Clara Demorest were students at the Kingston Women's Medical College. They both graduated in 1890. Elizabeth Mabel Henderson, also a K.W.M.C. student, graduated two years later. Billy Little consistently spelled Clara's name "Demerest," but K.W.M.C. records show it as "Demorest." She lived at Napanee (about 25 miles west of Kingston), so that is perhaps why a group of these students went there for what was obviously a memorable outing.

6. Laura B. Bennett, attended the K.W.M.C. from 1888 to 1891 but did not graduate. She had some serious intestinal illness and withdrew to her home in Windsor, Nova Scotia. History does not record the nature of her exciting yarn mentioned above.

7. Jessie (Nell) Savage was one of Grace Ritchie's three sisters.

8. Dr. Alice McGillivray was one of the three original women in medicine at the Royal. She was "Meshach" during the time of the male students' revolt. She was appointed to the K.W.M.C. immediately upon graduating in 1884, serving for five years as Professor of Obstetrics and Diseases of Women and Children. In 1889 she and her husband moved to Chicago.

9. Dr. Elizabeth Mitchell graduated from K.W.M.C. in 1888.

10. The Western Hospital, Montreal, where Dr. Grace Ritchie was later on staff.

11. Their landlord at the Kingston boarding house.

12. An extensive search through contemporary Montreal newspapers failed to uncover any of the details of this intriguing story.

13. Grace would be expected to take the qualifying exams of the Ontario Council of Physicians and Surgeons as well as those of the K.W.M.C.

14. Dr. James Allen Cross, who had been reading for the Licentiate of the Royal College of Surgeons in London. He was the one Grace thought "cheeky."

15. Dr. Chown was a medical practitioner in Kingston and lecturer at the K.W.M.C. He is also mentioned in Elizabeth Smith's diaries because he happened to be on hand on May 12, 1880, after the pioneer female medical students witnessed their first operation — the amputation of an old man's foot. Elizabeth Smith said, "Just before the finishing of it when I heard the joints parting company the foot go spat on the water, I felt kind o' sick and Miss Beaty and I left. I did not faint but was *very* white and weak. Soon after I went out — Oldham and Day came out to see if I had a fit or anything as that and out comes Mr. Mac and drops on the bed, dead sick. He did look bad to say the least. Dr. Day introduced Chown —B.A., M.D. to us. They took great satisfaction in staring at us and were glad I think that I was sick. I seemed quite an interesting monstrosity tho they were very kind. I'm bound to get over this — but oh it did leave me less strong than before. They say it is common for the men to faint — so I'm not so very bad."

16. Complained.

17. The other times would have been on the way to and from Ceylon.

18. Approximately $60. Until 1931 the Australian pound was at par with Sterling and worth $4.866 Canadian. W.C.L. usually converted from one currency to the other at the rate of $5 = £1.

19. Dr. William Joseph Cross had a medical practice at Horsham in the Western District of Victoria.

20. The group of female medical students in Kingston. "The Hen," "The Porpoise," "The Whale," etc.

21. January 16.

22. This picture of Victoria corresponds closely to the one by J.W. Springthorpe, M.A., M.D., M.R.C.P., Lecturer in Hygiene at the University of Melbourne in

a paper, "Hygiene Conditions in Victoria," given at the Intercolonial Medical Congress, 1889. See Diana J. Dyason, ed., "Glorious Smelbourne," History and Philosophy of Science Department, University of Melbourne, 1977, pp. 609–12.

23. William Brown was the Farm Manager and Professor of Livestock at the Ontario Agricultural College Guelph, when W.C.L. was a student there. Brown was in charge of the expedition to select livestock from Britain.

24. Grace was invited to enroll in the Faculty of Medicine of Bishop's College, which had hitherto been all male. She accepted the offer, regardless of W.C.L.'s reservations. However, he was at least partly right, for while Bishop's continues to thrive to this day, its Medical Faculty closed in 1905. Although it was the first institution in Quebec to offer medical training for women, it did so only for one decade and withdrew this opportunity for women five years before the Faculty of Medicine closed entirely.

25. This is one of the novels exerpted in the *Warracknabeal Herald*. Among other things, it has a highly enlightened view of the status of women in society. Grace certainly would have loved it.

26. Eight grains of quinine, four ounces of whiskey and Dover's Powder. The latter, named for English physician Thomas Dover (1660–1743), was a combination of ipecac and opium powder.

27. The Earl of Hopetoun was Governor of Victoria, 1889–1895.

28. Ammoniated copper.

29. Fellow of the Obstetrical Society, Edinburgh

30. Despite W.C.L.'s disapprobation of Trinity, his sister Isabella took her M.D. there in 1901. The reason for his low opinion is not known, for Trinity's reputation was and is deservedly high.

31. The 1891 Victorian census listed only one female physician.

32. For a discussion of this problem see Milton Lewis, "Doctors, Midwives, Puerperal Infection" in H. Attwood, Frank Forster, and B. Gardevia, eds., *Occasional Papers on Medical History of Australia*, Melbourne: Medical History Society, 1984, pp. 85–107.

33. Trichiasis — inverted eyelash; Entrofion — inner curling of the eyelid.

34. Wing-like structures, applied especially to a triangular fold of membrane extending, in the eye, from the conjunctiva to the cornea.

35. Pharez Phillips, a town councillor, was later (1901) elected as a member of the first parliament of the newly federated Commonwealth of Australia.

36. Maude Elizabeth Seymour Abbott was a close friend of Grace Ritchie in Montreal. She was an Arts graduate from McGill ('91) and then, like Grace, took her medical degree at Bishop's (Ch.M., M.D., '94). She won the Chancellor's gold medal on graduation. She later became world famous for her work on congenital heart disease.

37. Remove a circular disk of bone from the skull.

38. The following comments on W.C.L.'s prescriptions were supplied by Betty M. Plaskitt, Ph.C., M.P.S., J.P.:

No. 1
Chloroform 2 drachms
Creosote 32 minims
Peppermint Oil, 8-16 minims
Terebinth Oil, 16 minims–1 drachm
Menthol 8–16 grains
Cod liver oil to make volume 16 fluid ounces
Directions: 2 teasponsful 3 times daily after meals.
Acid Carbolic may be added to the above.

Comments: Extraordinary combination of medication for oral therapy, but I suppose phthisis (no doubt tuberculosis) was one of the most baffling of known complaints in those days.

My thoughts on his reasoning for presenting these ingredients:

Chloroform for its anaesthetic property; still used in gastric mixtures in form of Chloroform Water; 1/40 dilution.
Creosote for its decongestant property; still used for same reason in bronchial congestive complaints.
Peppermint Oil for its flavour and also to relieve digestive discomfort caused by accumulation of mucous. Still used as Peppermint Water — 1/40 dilution — in indigestion mixtures.
Terebinth Oil, i.e., Turpentine. I think this is more likely to be Terpin, which is an alcohol derived from turpentine and was used in treating lung diseases. Not used now.
Menthol for its dilation of bronchial tubes and so ease breathing. Only used now in inhalation for same reason.
Cod liver oil as a base for its therapeutic and prophylactic ingredients, vitamins A and D. Also the maintenance of body heat very necessary in such complaints. Still used in emulsion form as preventive medicine against colds and other kindred winter complaints and ailments.
Acid Carbolic — Carbolic Acid/Phenol. It would have to be used in miniscule quantity owing to its caustic property. Maybe internal cauterization was the object. If mixed initially with the Menthol and the resultant solution added to the mixture, the corrosive property is diminished.

Final comment: No wonder the Chinaman died in four hours!

No.2
Alcohol (90% Rectified Spirit); Solution of Nutgal. (Nutgal is extract from insects' eggs on oak tree.) 5 fluid oz.
Menthol, 8 grains.
Tincture of iodine 24 minims.
Glycerine to volume 12 fluid oz.

Directions: 2 teaspoonsful increased to 4 teaspoonsful (i.e., one tablespoon three times daily).

My thoughts on ingredients can only be educated guesses: Spt. Nutgal for astringent property; Menthol for same reason as in first prescription; Tincture Iodine, I think this is not the tincture *per se* but rather a solution, the former being an alcoholic preparation 10% iodine crystals. The latter is a much weaker aqueous solution especially for oral medication and commonly called Lugels Iodine. It is *very* rarely used now but enjoyed considerable popularity for abdominal problems, suspected appendix in particular, and also for thyroid problems; Glycerine for its soothing warmth on the throat and chest — still used as an ingredient in cough linctus.

"Paint chest with iodine": This could be for the absorption through the skin of the tincture of iodine to combat a condition that could well have been scabies, which would not be surprising in those debilitated patients.

"Combination of glycerine, brandy, menthol" would be for reasons already stated, with the addition of brandy as a painkiller in the advanced stages. There are two standard formulae still *very* occasionally used in advanced carcinoma, containing brandy or whiskey and cocaine in a syrup base.

"Ol. Murrhuae, Spts. Turpentine, Chloroform and Menthol Combined": This is a repeat of prescription no. 1.

39. Dr. James Allen Cross, who had previously been in London. He later settled in Murtoa, not far from Warracknabeal.

40. Constance Stone had attempted to register for Medicine at the University of Melbourne but was not accepted because of her sex. She left in 1884 to study at the Women's Medical College in Philadelphia and did post-graduate work in Toronto. Her sister Clara became one of the first two female medical graduates at the University of Melbourne. See Farley Kelly, *Degrees of Liberation: A Short History of the University of Melbourne,* 1985, p. 15.

41. No trace of Shuttleworth can be found in either the Royal's or Queen's graduating lists.

42. After Robert James Graves, Irish physician, 1797–1853; exophthalmic goiter.

43. Probably Narcisse G. Cantin, who graduated in Medicine from Bishop's in 1894.

44. Grace apparently contemplated conversion to Roman Catholicism from Methodism, but she did not take this step.

45. The letter clearly says $500, i.e., he had converted pounds to dollars. The actually salary was £50 initially, then £100.

46. Sir John A. Macdonald (1815–1891) became Canada's first prime minister in 1867. He was defeated in the 1872 election but returned to power in 1878 and was prime minister for the rest of his life.

47. When the placenta is implanted in the lower third of the uterus and partially or completely occludes the os or opening of the uterus.

48. Whooping cough.

49. "Whitlow" or suppurative inflammation of the upper part of the finger.

50. Grace was presumably using this classic mixture as a skin toner for her complexion.

51. Painful swelling of the leg caused by a clot or infection in a major vein.

52. Chloroform.

53. Uncoordinated movement due to the posterior roots of the spinal cord. Its most common cause in the nineteenth century was syphilis and the ataxia was very often accompanied by "lightening pains" that were very intense and of sudden onset and disappearance.

54. A rare hereditary disease of the spine and spinal cord; unrelated to syphilis.

55. A phenol derived from wood creosote, which had been a popular medication since the fifteenth century and was still extensively used in the nineteenth century.

56. Osteitis or cares of the vertebrae, usually of tuberculous origin.

57. W.C.L.'s sister Isabella graduated in Medicine from Trinity College, University of Toronto in 1901. She went to China as a medical missionary, married Dr. I. Mitchell of Hong Kong, but later contracted typhoid and died in Canton in 1905.

PART IV — "AND SO THEY LIVED . . ."

1. Letter from H.J. Hackett, medical secretary, The Western Hospital to Dr. G. Ritchie-England, January 13, 1906.

2. Letter from Geo. T. Roper, Hon. Sec., The Western Hospital to Dr. Grace Ritchie-England, January 20, 1906.

3. Mrs. Warwick Chipman, "An Address to Dr. Grace Ritchie-England, B.A.," Montreal, December 27, 1918, p. 3.

4. Esther England Cushing, "I Remember, I Remember, . . ." in Margaret Gillett and Kay Sibbald, eds., *A Fair Shake: Autobiographical Essays by McGill Women,* Montreal: Eden Press, 1984, p. 191.

5. "Mrs. Dr. Ritchie-England endorses Sir Wilfrid Laurier," political pamphlet, Montreal, December 6, 1917.

6. "Woman's Club Splits Over Free Speech," *Montreal Star,* February 20, 1918, p. 1.

7. Mrs. Warwick Chipman, "An Address . . . ," p. 1; see also "Presentation to Dr. Grace Ritchie England," *Sherbrooke Standard,* December 28, 1918, n.p.

8. "Result Satisfied Dr. G.R. England — Feminist Movement Aided by Choice of Woman as Official Candidate," *The Gazette,* Montreal, July 30, 1930.

9.   See Dorothy Green, *Ulysses Bound,* Canberra: Australian National University Press, 1973, p. 382. Green notes that "Spiritualism emerged in the United States in the 1840's and swept through Northern Europe in the late sixties and seventies. A ripple of its wave reached the shores of Victoria in the 50's and gathered strength in 1869 when Dr. Walter Richardson became the first President of the Victorian Association for Progressive Spiritualists," p. 86.

10.   Full accounts of the Jewitt and Logan cases can be found in the reports of the regular monthly and special meetings of the hospital committee in the *Warracknabeal Herald,* 1901. Commentary and letters to the editor appeared in the *Northern Argus* during the year.

11.   Marion Steel, "Introductory Notes to Aunt Jenny's Diaries," p. 1, n.d.

12.   Extract from letter from Iris Darling to Daisy Searby, Warracknabeal, September 26, 1964. Original in possession of Mrs. G. Steel, Frankson, Victoria.

13.   Gwen Steel, "The Steel Family," Frankson, Victoria, February, 1965, pp. 17–18.

14.   Susan Priestly, *Warracknabeal — A Wimmera Centenary,* Brisbane and Melbourne: Jacaranda Press, 1967, p. 84.

SOURCES

As can be seen from the text, much information and insight came from conversations, interviews and correspondence. The written sources used in the project included the following:

Adam Shortt Papers, Queen's University Archives

Attwood, H., F. Foster and B. Gandevia, eds. *Occasional Papers on Medical History in Australia*. Melbourne: Medical History Society, University of Melbourne, 1984.

Australia, Department of Labor and Immigration. *1788-1975 — Australia and Immigration*. Canberra: Australia Government Service, 1975.

Barrie Examiner (*The*).

Blainey, Geoffrey. *A Land Half Won*. Melbourne: Sun Books, 1983.

Brown, Frances, Dom Meadley, Marjorie Morgan. *Family and Local History Sources in Victoria*. Blackburn: Custodian of Records, 1983.

Bruck, Ludwig. *On the Uses and Abuses of the Public Hospitals in Australia, Tasmania and New Zealand*. Sydney: Bruck, 1899.

Bruck, Ludwig, compiler. *The Australasian Medical Directory*. Sydney: Bruck, 1883, 1886, 1892, 1896.

Cage, R.A. *The Scots Abroad: Labour, Capital, Enterprise 1750-1914*. London: Croom Helm, 1985.

Calendar of the Kingston Women's Medical College in Affiliation with Queen's University, 1884-85. Kingston: The College, 1884.

Calendar of the Royal College of Physicians and Surgeons in Affiliation with Queen's University. Kingston: The College, 1884-1889.

Canadian Medical Association. *Journal*, 1889-1912.

Canniff, William. *The Medical Profession in Upper Canada, 1783-1850*. Toronto: Hannah Institute, 1980. (First published 1894).

Cleverdon, Catherine L. *The Woman Suffrage Movement in Canada*. Toronto: University of Toronto Press, 1950.

Dunmunkle Standard (Murtoa), 1911.

Dyason, Diana J., compiler. *Glorious Smelbourne — Health, Hygiene and History*. Melbourne: Department of History and Philosophy of Science, University of Melbourne, 1977.

Edwards, William. *Mesmerism: Its Practice and Phenomena*. Melbourne: John Hunter, 1850.

Fleming, W.G. *Ontario's Educative Society — IV — "Post Secondary and Adult Education."* Toronto: University of Toronto, 1971.

Ford, Edward. *Bibliography of Australian Medicine.* Sydney: Sydney University Press, 1976.

Gaff, Janet Muir Steel. *Diaries*, unpublished, 1910-11.

General Report on the Census on Victoria, taken on the 5th April, 1891 . . . by the Government Statistician. Melbourne: Government Printer, 1893.

Gillett, Margaret. *We Walked Very Warily: A History of Women at McGill.* Montreal: Eden Press, 1981.

Gillett, Margaret and Kay Sibbald, eds. *A Fair Shake: Autobiographical Essays by McGill Women.* Montreal: Eden Press, 1984.

Godfrey, Charles M. "The Evolution of Medical Education in Ontario." University of Toronto, unpublished M.A. Thesis, 1974.

Grace Ritchie-England Papers (courtesy Mrs. Esther Cushing).

Green, Dorothy. *Ulysses Bound.* Canberra: Australian National University Press, 1973.

Green, Dorothy. "Walter Lindesay Richardson: The Man, the Portrait, the Artist." *Meanjin* 1/70.

Grove, Abraham. *All in the Day's Work: Leaves from a Doctor's Case Book.* Toronto: Macmillan, 1934.

Gundy, H.P. "Growing Pains: The Early History of Queen's Medical Faculty," *Historic Kingston*, No. 4 (1954-5). pp. 14-25.

Hacker, Carlotta. *The Indomitable Lady Doctors.* Toronto: Clarke, Irwin & Co., 1974.

Historical Atlas of Simcoe County, Ontario, H. Belden & Co., 1881.

Innis, Mary Quayle. *Unfold the Years. A History of the Young Women's Christian Association in Canada.* Toronto: McClelland & Stewart, 1949.

Keane, David Ross. "Rediscovering Ontario Students of the Mid-Nineteeth Century: Sources for and Approaches to the Study of the Experience of Going to College and Personal, Family and Social Backgrounds of Students." University of Toronto, unpublished Ph.D. thesis, 1981. 4 vols.

Kelley, Farley. *Degrees of Liberation. A Short History of Women in the University of Melbourne.* Melbourne: Women Graduates' Centennary Committee, University of Melbourne, 1985.

Leitch, Adelaide. *The Visible Past. The Pictorial History of Simcoe County.* County of Simcoe, 1967.

Little, William C. *Last Will and Testament.* Public Records Office of Victoria, 127/949, p.227. (February 11, 1911).

Loh, Morag. "Victoria as a Catalyst for Western and Chinese Medicine," *Journal*, Royal Historical Society of Melbourne, Vol. 56, No. 3(September 1985), pp.38-46.

MacLean, George, ed. *The Canadian Cyclopaedia of Biography.* Toronto: Rose Publishing, 1886.

MacSporran, Maysie S. "Vale, Amica Carissima," *The McGill News*, Spring 1948, n.p.

Matthews, R.M. "Philosophy of the Fee Schedule," *Ontario Medical Review*, Vol. 31(1964), pp.21-23.

"Medical Officers and Hospital Committees," *The Australasian Medical Gazette*, June 29, 1912, p.687 ff.

Montreal Gazette (The).

Montreal Herald (The).

Montreal Star (The).

Northern Argus (Warracknabeal).

Ontario Agricultural College. *Annual Reports*, Guelph: The College, 1882-84.

Priestly, Susan. *Warracknabeal — A Wimmera Centenary*. Brisbane and Melbourne: Jacaranda Press, 1967.

Queen's College Journal, 1884-1890.

Racster, Olga and Jessica Grove. *Dr. James Barry: Her Secret Story*. London: Gerald Howe, 1932.

Rate Book, Borung Shire (Warracknabeal), 1891-1937.

Record of 100 Years of Progress: Innisfil Township Centennial 1850-1950 — Historical Review. Barrie: Innisfil Township Council, 1951.

Richardson, Henry Handel. *The Fortunes of Richard Mahony*. Ringwood, Vic.: Penguin, 1982 (First published 1930).

Rosen, George. "Fees and Fee Bills: Some Economic Aspects of Medical Practice in 19th Century America," *History of Medicine Bulletin*, Supplement No. 6. Baltimore: Johns Hopkins, 1947.

Sherbrooke Standard (The).

Shortt, Elizabeth Smith. *Historical Sketch of Medical Education of Women, Kingston, Canada*. Ottawa: Private Printing, 1916.

Smith, Elizabeth (Shortt). *A Woman with a Purpose: The Diaries of Elizabeth Smith 1872-1884*. Edited, with an introduction, by Veronica Strong-Boag. Toronto: University of Toronto Press, 1980.

Steel, Gwenyth. *The Steel Family*. Frankston, Vic.: Private Printing, 1965.

Stoller, Alan and R.H. Emerson, "The Fortunes of Walter Lindesay Richardson," *Meanjin Quarterly*, No. 1, 1970, pp.21-33.

Travill, A.A. "Early Medical Co-Education: Women's Medical College, Kingston, Ontario, 1880-1894." *Historic Kingston*, Vol. 30 (January 1982), pp.68-89.

"Warracknabeal" in *The Cyclopedia of Victoria*. Melbourne: 1905, Vol. III, pp.249-258.

"Warracknabeal" in *The Victorian Municipal Directory and Gazeteer*. Melbourne: Arnall and Jackson, 1890.

Warracknabeal and N.W. Advertiser, 1908-11.

Warracknabeal Herald, 1889-1911.

Warunda Review, Warracknabeal Historial Society Bulletin, 1982.

"William Clow Little," in *The Cyclopedia of Victoria*, Melbourne: 1905, Vol. III, pp. 252-3.